Making Healthy Decisions
Fitness

Unit 1

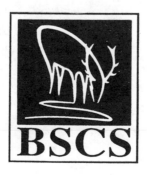

BSCS

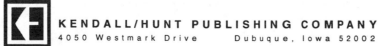

KENDALL/HUNT PUBLISHING COMPANY
4050 Westmark Drive   Dubuque, Iowa 52002

ADVISORY COMMITTEE
Lawrence W. Green
Donald C. Iverson
Lloyd J. Kolbe
Nathan Maccoby
Katharine G. Sommers

BSCS PROJECT STAFF
Nancy M. Landes, Project Director and Revision
Coordinator, Final Edition
James D. Ellis, Project Director, Field-test Edition
Rodger W. Bybee, Contributing Author
Joseph D. McInerney, Contributing Author
Susan Frelick Wooley, Contributing Author
Teresa T. Hendrickson, Editor, Field-test Edition
C. Yvonne Wise, Editor, Final Edition
Jan Girard, Art Coordinator
Byllee Simon, Senior Executive Assistant

WRITING TEAMS, FIELD-TEST EDITIONS
Katherine A. Corley, Middle School Teacher
Sandra L.H. Davenport, M.D.
Ann Junk, Middle School Teacher
Terry Shaw, Middle School Teacher
David R. Stronck, Health Educator
Gordon Thies, Health Educator
Gordon E. Uno, Science Educator

REVIEWERS, FIELD-TEST EDITIONS
Steven N. Blair
Glen Gilbert
Gilda Gussin
Louise Light
Peter D. Loranger
Richard R.J. Lauzon
Terry Shaw
David A. Sleet

BSCS ADMINISTRATIVE STAFF
Timothy H. Goldsmith, Chair, Board of Directors
Joseph D. McInerney, Director
Lawrence Satkowiak, Chief Financial Officer

FIELD-TEST SCHOOLS
Challenger Middle School, Colorado Springs,
Colorado
Aspen Middle School, Aspen, Colorado
Buffalo Ridge Elementary School, Grade 6,
Laramie, Wyoming
Calhan Elementary School, Grade 6, Calhan,
Colorado
Carver Elementary School, Grade 6, Colorado
Springs, Colorado
Kearney Middle School, Commerce City,
Colorado
Ortega Middle School, Alamosa, Colorado
Sabin Junior High School, Colorado Springs,
Colorado
Sproul Junior High School, Widefield, Colorado
Webster Elementary School, Grade 6, Widefield,
Colorado
Widefield Elementary School, Grade 6, Widefield,
Colorado
Watson Junior High School, Widefield, Colorado

ARTISTS/PHOTOGRAPHERS
Susan Bartle
Brenda Bundy
Carlye Calvin
Jan Girard
Nancy Smalls
Linn Trochim

ISBN 0-7872-1222-9

This work was supported by the Gates Foundation, the Helen K. and Arthur E. Johnson Foundation, the Piton
Foundation, and the Adolph Coors Foundation. However, the opinions expressed herein do not necessarily reflect
the position or policies of the funding agencies, and no official endorsement should be inferred.

10 9 8 7 6 5 4 3 2 1

TABLE OF CONTENTS

UNIT 1: FITNESS

FOREWORD

Whether you are aware of it or not, you make decisions about your health all day, every day. You are making decisions about your health when you decide what to eat for breakfast or whether to eat breakfast at all, whether to brush and floss your teeth, whether to wear a safety belt if you ride to school in a car, how to communicate with your classmates and teachers once you arrive at school, what to eat for lunch, whether to participate in sports or exercise after school, which television programs you watch, and when you go to sleep. Believe it or not, just about everything you do has some impact on your health and YOU are in charge of most of those decisions. Are the decisions you make healthy ones? How do you know? Do you care?

Sometimes, it's tough to make healthy decisions. All of us have lots of excuses: It's not what my friends are doing. I'm not sick, so why worry about what I eat? I'm careful, so I'm not going to get hurt. I really don't have time to exercise. No one else in the car has on a safety belt. In the lessons you are about to experience, we hope to convince you that it makes sense to pay attention to your health while you're healthy. Although some of the actions you take might not have an effect until years later, many decisions will make a difference right now in how you feel, how you relate to your friends and family, whether or not you become injured, whether you contract a life-threatening illness, or whether you put someone else's life and health at risk.

We sincerely hope you enjoy the activities in this unit of *Making Healthy Decisions* and that they make a difference in how you care for yourself and those around you. Remember, the healthy decisions are up to you.

Nancy M. Landes
Revision Director

James D. Ellis
Project Director
Field-test Edition

INTRODUCTION TO FITNESS

What does physical fitness mean to you? According to the President's Council on Physical Fitness and Sports, a fit person is one who:

has the energy and strength to perform daily activities vigorously and alertly without getting "run down," and

has energy left over to enjoy leisure-time activities and meet emergency demands.

Do you meet those guidelines? Do you participate in some type of vigorous physical activity, such as brisk walking, jogging, swimming, basketball, or soccer, at least three times a week?

Being fit can be fun for everyone. You don't have to be an athlete or be "the best" to become fit, but you do have to be active and participate in some form of physical activity at least three times a week. Through the lessons in this unit, you will experience the benefits of fitness and determine your current level of fitness. By working out with your classmates, you can improve your level of fitness and have fun at the same time. Becoming physically fit doesn't require special skills or athletic abilities. YOU can do it!

Personal health is not something you can take for granted. Investing in fitness is one way to gain big health benefits, both now and in the future. Not only will you look better as you "shape up," but you will feel great and have more energy to enjoy the things you like to do.

Becoming more active is a healthy decision you can make. Get up off that couch, turn off the TV, and get moving. It's up to you to make fitness fun!

BELIEVE IT OR NOT

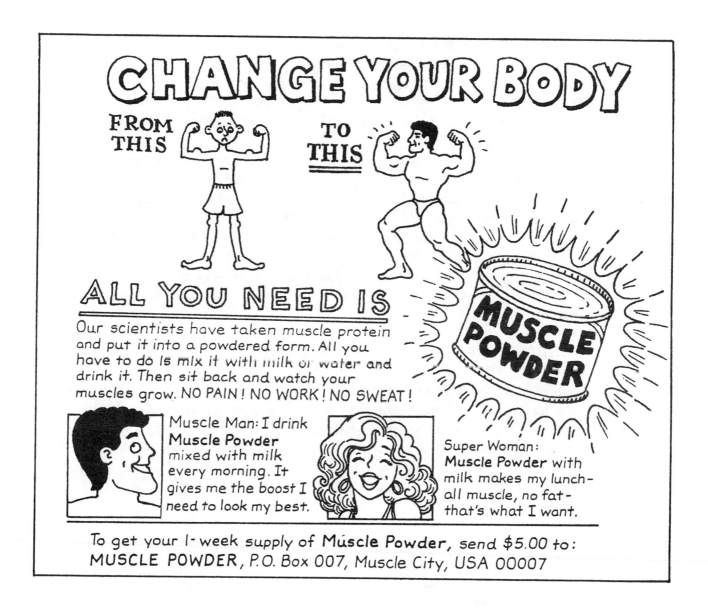

Wow, Muscle Powder! Just what I've been waiting for. One quick fix and I won't even have to sweat. I can't wait to get my hands on some of that stuff. It sounds too good to be true.

Stop and think. If it sounds too good to be true, is it too good to be true? Do you believe the claims made in the advertisement for Muscle Powder? Take a closer look.

ACTIVITY: DO YOU BELIEVE THE AD?

Procedure

1. Reread the advertisement for Muscle Powder.
2. Write your answers to the following questions:
    Why do you think people believe ads that promise quick and easy methods for self-improvement?
    How could you investigate whether Muscle Powder works? (Would you have to try it for yourself?)
    Are there any clues in the ad that would help you decide whether to try Muscle Powder?
3. With a partner or in a team, discuss your answers to the questions.
4. Read and discuss the information in the following two readings: "Direct Versus Indirect Evidence" and "Looking for Clues in Advertisements."
5. Review your team's answers to the questions from Step 3. Write a team answer for each question, adding any new information you found in the two readings.
    You could simply combine all your answers or write new answers to the questions based on your discussion. Share the writing task so that one team member doesn't have to do all of the writing.

READING: DIRECT VERSUS INDIRECT EVIDENCE

Sometimes, when you investigate the solutions to problems or the answers to questions, you use your senses and make personal observations. Sometimes, you might expand your senses by using tools, such as telescopes or thermometers. When you directly use your senses (with or without appropriate tools) to gather evidence, that evidence is called **direct evidence**. Many scientists gather direct evidence about the world around us and products we might use by making observations and conducting tests in a laboratory or "in the field." But, is it always safe to gather direct evidence by using your senses and making personal observations with or without proper tools?

There are other ways to get evidence. One way is to listen to or read about what other people have observed. For example, do you have to smoke cigarettes yourself to find out that cigarette smoking causes lung cancer in many people? No, you can use **indirect evidence** reported by scientists and medical researchers who have studied the effects of cigarette smoking in those people who do smoke.

When you consider indirect evidence from other people, you should ask questions. Do not believe everything you read or hear. Some questions you might ask are

4

Who is the person providing the evidence? Does the person have special training in this area? Does the person have experience in this area?

How does the person know? Did the person investigate the problem and make direct observations? What evidence does the person give? (It is not evidence if people make claims based on what they believe rather than on what they observe.) Also, if people make claims based on only one person's experience, look for more evidence.

Are the person's explanations based on the observations? Do the explanations or claims make sense to you? If the person does not give evidence, are there ways to test the claims? How might the claims be tested?

Finally, remember that even the experts are wrong sometimes, or at least they do not always agree. That is part of the scientific process. You have probably heard about the importance of "getting a second opinion." This recommendation also is important in gathering information and evidence. You should always read the evidence and conclusions from more than one expert before you make up your mind about a problem or question.

READING: LOOKING FOR CLUES IN ADVERTISEMENTS

You have thought about ways to investigate the claims made in advertisements. There are some common clues that can help you decide whether to believe the ad's claims. Some clues should tell you to

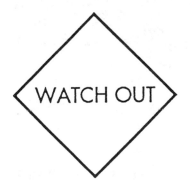 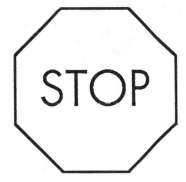 

When you look at advertisements, you should ask questions.

Where does the ad appear? (Which would probably be more reliable: an ad in a comic book or an ad in a scientific journal?)

What evidence does the ad present? Is the evidence based on someone's observations and investigations or on an individual's stories? Does the ad sell an image or a product?

Will the people who gave evidence benefit if you buy the product or service?

How reliable is the company selling the product? Does the company's address include a building or an office location, or just a post office box number?

Does the claim make sense to you? Are the changes the ad promises possible? Is the ad believable?

ACTIVITY: WHAT ARE THE CLUES?

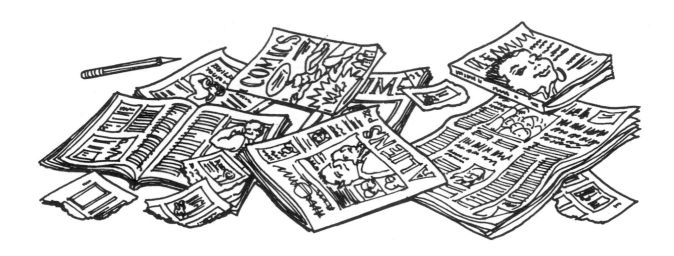

Procedure

1. From magazines, comic books, or newspapers, collect advertisements of products or services that promise a beautiful body or ways to "improve" the body. Bring the ads to class.
   You could also videotape ads from the television and bring those to class.
2. With a partner or as a team, examine the ads you and your teammates brought to school. Find clues that help you decide whether to believe the claims in the ads.
3. Make a list of the clues the team thinks would help to evaluate the claims made in the ads.
4. Look at one advertisement at a time, and decide as a team whether to believe the claims made in that particular ad.

5.   Share your conclusions about the advertisements with your classmates.

Stop and Discuss

1.   Why is it important to examine advertisements before you buy a product or use a service?
2.   Why do you think this lesson about reading advertisements is in a unit about physical fitness?

WRAP UP

Review the claims made in the ad for Muscle Powder. Discuss with your classmates ways you could change your body if you wanted to have stronger muscles or look better without using something like Muscle Powder. List those ways of changing your body on the board or on a chart.

Make an advertisement for one of those methods of improving your body through physical fitness. How can you make your advertisement appealing? How can you base your advertisement on evidence?

INVOLVING FAMILY MEMBERS

With your parents or guardians, look at advertisements for products or services in the newspaper or magazines. (These can be advertisements for any type of product or service.) Ask them whether they would buy the product or service and their reasons for their answer. Then, share with them what you learned about reading ads carefully and looking for claims and evidence to back up those claims. Do you agree with your parents or guardians about how to choose products or services from ads? Why or why not?

WHAT IS FITNESS?

Remember Muscle Powder? Here's someone who just might go for it. Or, will he listen to his friend's advice?

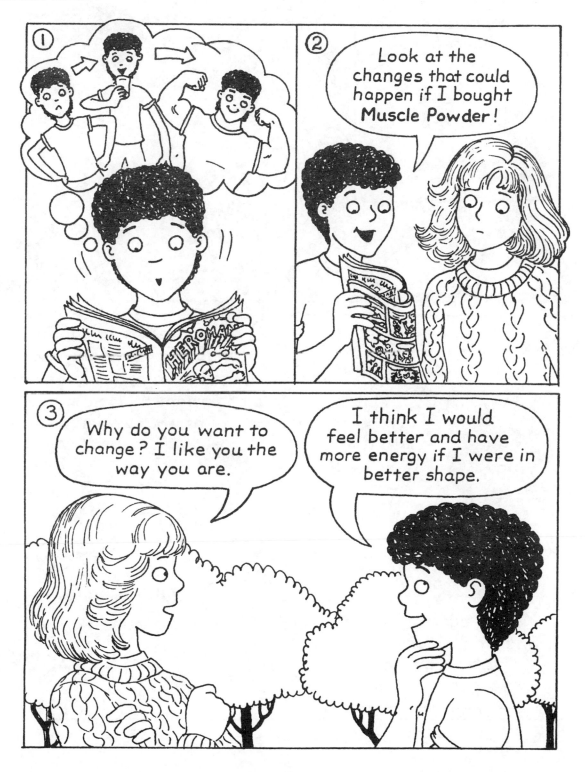

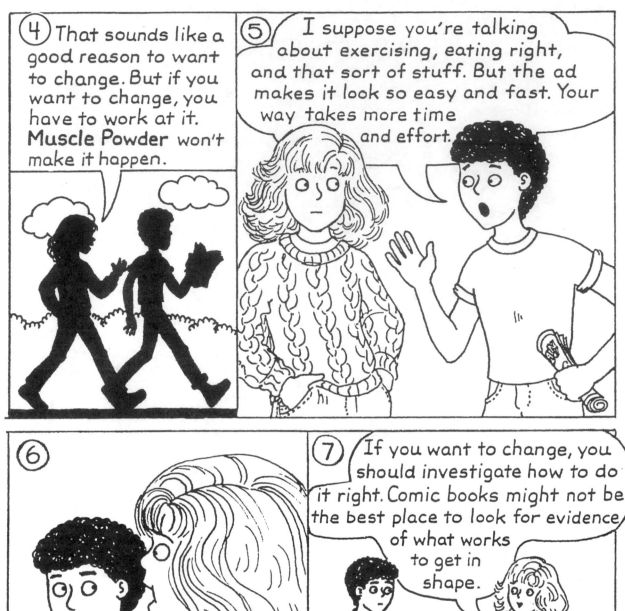

READING: MAKING CHANGES

Many people wish they could change something about themselves. Sometimes, people want to change because, although they like themselves, they want to make themselves better. They might want to change something about themselves, but not who they are. When these people decide to change themselves, they usually feel good about the changes they make. Sometimes, people want to change because they do not like themselves and want to be something or somebody else. They want to change who or what they are. When these people decide to change, they usually are disappointed with the results. They might make the changes, but they still have the same problems.

Think about the changes you want in your life. You might consider whether those changes would really do what you hope they would do. If you are unsure, talk to others about your ideas. You might be surprised that what you think is a big problem that requires change is actually something that no one else even notices.

Think about answers to the following questions. The answers are only for you. You will not share them with others.

- What would you like to change about how you live?
- What would you like to change about how you act?
- What would you like to change about how you look?
- Do you want to make these changes to please yourself or to please others?

Changes that some people make for themselves include getting enough sleep, spending more time with friends, eating foods that provide the nutrients the body needs without a lot of fat, laughing more, crying when they feel like crying, undertaking a new project, trying a new hairstyle, and exercising regularly.

In this unit, you will learn some ways you can become more fit. As you go through the unit, think about how you feel about becoming more fit. Think about whether becoming more fit is a change you would like to make for yourself.

ACTIVITY: WHAT DO YOU KNOW ABOUT FITNESS?

You have no doubt heard the term "physical fitness." What does physical fitness mean to you? Are you involved or on the sidelines? In this lesson, you will define physical fitness for yourself and decide how you can get started.

Procedure

1. As a class, brainstorm everything you know that has to do with physical fitness. Record your ideas on chart paper and post them so that you can see them every day.
   Make your list as long as possible. Include things on your list that might not seem directly related, such as getting enough sleep at night.

2.   On a sheet of paper, make two columns: Things I Already Do to Become Fit and Things I Would Like to Do to Become More Fit.
This will be a personal list; you do not need to share it with anyone else. Save your list, though, because you will need it later in the unit.

3.   Now, as a class, brainstorm all the benefits of becoming physically fit. Record your ideas and post them with your ideas about physical fitness.
You will add to this list as the unit progresses.

ACTIVITY: BECOMING FIT

You cannot become fit by sitting around. Let's get busy! Your teacher will lead you in a workout for physical fitness. As you go through the activities and exercises, pay attention to how your body feels. Which muscles are working? Does your breathing rate change or stay the same? What happens to your heart beats? How do you feel when the workout is over? Remember to work at your own pace. This is not a contest, but a "fitness experience." Have fun.

READING: DEFINING FITNESS

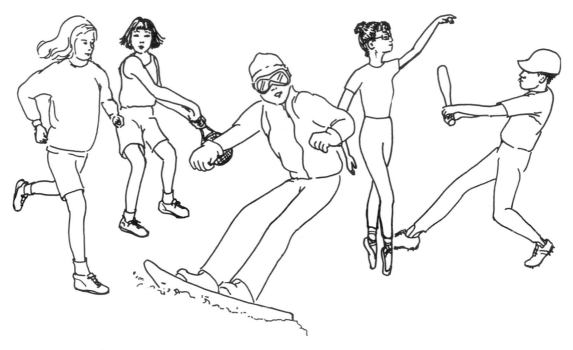

The President's Council on Physical Fitness and Sports says a fit person is one who:

●   has the energy and strength to perform daily activities vigorously and alertly without getting "run down," and

●   has energy left over to enjoy leisure-time activities and meet emergency demands.

That is not a very specific definition. "Daily activities" and "leisure-time activities" can be very different for each of us. It is very hard to give an answer to the question, "How fit should I be?"

Each of us should be fit enough to do the things that we normally do without getting overly tired. Also, we should be able to participate in light activities and respond to emergencies without risking injury.

We cannot say *exactly* how fit each of us should be. Yet experts know that overall fitness is a combination of many things, such as

- exercising regularly,
- maintaining moderate weight,
- eating breakfast,
- eating well-balanced meals,
- not snacking between meals,
- avoid smoking, and
- sleeping at least seven to eight hours each night.

In this unit, you will be looking mainly at the relationship between exercise and physical fitness. You will learn about four types of physical fitness: cardiovascular fitness, muscular strength, muscular endurance, and flexibility. Each is developed by different activities and exercises.

Cardiovascular fitness is the most essential part of physical fitness. "Cardio" means heart, "vascular" means the blood vessels. This type of fitness helps the heart and blood vessels move oxygen in the blood to all parts of the body. It also helps the lungs supply oxygen to the blood. Activities that improve cardiovascular fitness are often called aerobic activities. In aerobic activities, the heart rate and breathing rate increase. Activities that improve cardiovascular fitness include running, swimming, bicycling, cross-country skiing, jumping rope, and aerobic dancing. To improve cardiovascular fitness, aerobic exercise should last at least 15 minutes without stopping. To keep fit, a person should do some type of aerobic activity at least three times a week.

When you have cardiovascular endurance, you will not get out of breath as quickly as you would if you were not fit. Having a fit heart reduces a person's chances of having heart attacks and strokes—two major killers of adults. Aerobic exercise—exercise that builds cardiovascular endurance—also helps control the amount of fat on a person's body. Aerobic exercise uses a lot of energy.

Muscular strength is the area most often associated with physical fitness. People often think that if someone has big, well-defined muscles, then that person must be physically fit. However, muscular strength is only **one** component of fitness. Someone can have big muscles and not be very fit, and a fit person can have strong muscles without having them bulge. Muscular strength can be measured by how much weight you can lift, push, or pull. To increase strength, you must provide resistance to the muscles. You could provide resistance to the muscles by lifting weights, for example, or by pushing up your body weight in push-ups, or by pulling up your body weight in chin-ups. It is important to develop strong muscles in all parts of the body, but especially in the abdomen and upper body. A person needs abdominal and upper-body strength to have good posture and to avoid injuries to the lower back.

Muscular endurance is not the same as muscular strength. Endurance is the ability of the muscles to do the same motion over and over again for increasing periods of time. When you have muscular endurance, you can work and play for a long time and your muscles will not get tired. The number of curl-ups or pull-ups you can do is related to your muscular endurance. How long you can shovel snow, hit a tennis ball, wash windows, or jog is due to your muscular (and cardiovascular) endurance, not just strength.

Flexibility is a measure of how far you can move the joints and muscles in your body, such as your knees and shoulders and your back, arm, and leg muscles. Flexibility exercises improve the range of motion of the joints. Activities such as gymnastics increase flexibility. Those activities stretch the muscles gradually and involve bending and stretching. Stretching is a very important part of exercising. Proper stretching before and after a strenuous workout helps avoid injuries and soreness. Flexibility also reduces injuries. Joint movement and stretching exercises improve flexibility and help relieve tension and stress.

All the components of fitness help to maintain a lean body, which does not always mean a small, thin body. A lean body does not have extra fat. Extra fat makes the body work harder. Moving the extra weight takes energy. Regular exercise builds muscles and uses energy and will help make your body firm. (By the way, people can have extra fat without looking fat if they do not have good muscle tone. Someone can be large and still be lean. It all depends on how fit a person is. Size is not the issue.)

A workout program to increase total fitness must include all four components of fitness. One way to set up a total workout plan is, as follows:

1.   Warm-up (flexibility) — minimum 5 minutes (recommended time: 10 minutes every time you exercise)

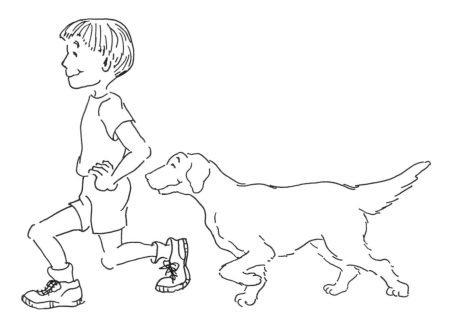

The warm-up gets you ready for more strenuous exercise. You should include stretching exercises that use all the major joints and muscles. You should use the full range of motion of each joint. Move your joints all around. As your muscles warm up, they stretch. Then, they are less likely to get injured. Stretching should be smooth, so do not bounce when you are stretching. Move from stretching to light, rhythmical exercises. Move slowly at first, gradually getting faster. The movement that warms up muscles starts the heart beating faster. As you move faster, your heart rate will get faster, too. Then your heart is ready for a harder workout.

2.   Cardiovascular Fitness (aerobic activity) — minimum 15 minutes (recommended time: 20 to 30 minutes, three days a week)

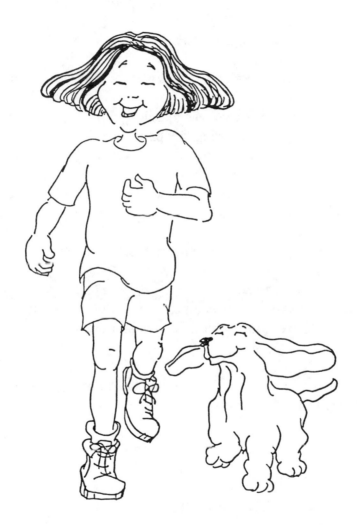

Aerobic activity improves cardiovascular fitness. In the lessons to follow, you will learn how to do some aerobic exercises that will make your heart beat faster and cause you to breathe harder. You must continue aerobic activity at an increased heart rate for at least 15 minutes each time you exercise.

3.   Muscular Strength and Endurance — minimum 5 minutes (recommended time: 10 minutes, 2 to 3 times a week)

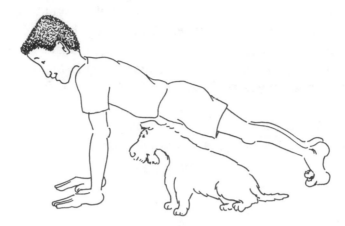

This part of the workout should provide resistance to all the major muscles of your abdomen, legs, and arms. Those exercises will help to increase strength. Do not spend too much time on one muscle group. Your breathing and heart rate should not increase too much during this part of the workout. It is not a good idea to do one exercise until you are exhausted. Instead do a set of five to eight repetitions, or "reps." Then rest. Do another set, rest, and so on. Three or four sets should be enough for each group of muscles. Remember, do not bounce or move in jerky motions. Move smoothly.

After a few days, increase the number of times you do each exercise. Continue to increase the number of times you do each exercise over many days. Once an exercise becomes easy to do ten times, make the exercise harder. Add weight, or resistance, but do the exercise fewer times. Be careful not to work your muscles too hard so that you are sore. Sometimes, people who get sore muscles get discouraged and stop exercising.

4.   Cool-down (flexibility) — minimum 5 minutes (recommended time: 10 minutes every time you exercise)

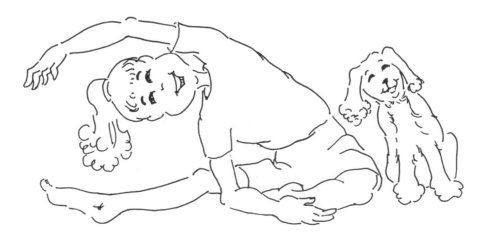

The cool-down period gives your muscles time to rebuild energy. Start by doing the aerobic exercises more slowly or by walking. Then, do some stretching, or flexibility, exercises. Now that your muscles are warmed up, they will stretch farther than they did at the beginning of the exercise period. Do stretches slowly and hold each position for a few seconds. Stretching as a cool-down exercise will help prevent soreness later. As you do your cool-down exercises, gradually slow down, so your pulse rate will slow down. The cool-down period will help you relax, too.

Stop and Discuss

1. Describe a workout that would provide all four parts of fitness. Does that workout sound like fun to you?
2. How might you make fitness fun for you and your friends?

ACTIVITY: COUNTING YOUR PULSE

Every time your heart muscles contract, your heart pumps blood through your body. Blood travels through the blood vessels to all parts of your body. Arteries carry blood from your heart through your body, and veins carry the blood from your body back to your heart.

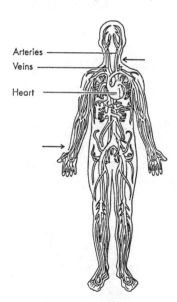

Arteries

Veins

Heart

Some of your arteries are near the surface of the skin where you can feel the blood pulsing through them. Each time you feel a pulse, or a beat, your heart has contracted. The number of times your artery pulses in one minute is called your **pulse rate**. Your pulse rate is the same as your heart rate.

When you exercise to improve your cardiovascular fitness, you will need to measure your exercising pulse rate. Follow the procedure and learn to measure your pulse rate as accurately as possible.

Procedure

1. Look at the following drawings that show two ways you can measure your pulse.
   Notice that you can measure your pulse at either your wrist or at the side of your neck.

2. Because the pulse in the side of the neck is stronger and easier to find, try that first. Place the flat part of two fingers in the hollow spot at the side of your neck, just under your chin and above your Adam's apple. (See Figure 2.8.) Press in lightly.
   You can use your right hand to feel a pulse on the right side of your neck or your left hand to feel a pulse on the left side of your neck. Be sure to use your fingertips and not your thumb to find your pulse. Your thumb has a tiny pulse of its own and might confuse your counting. Don't press too hard. If you can't feel your pulse right away, move your fingers around on that part of your neck until you feel a slight "jump" in the artery.

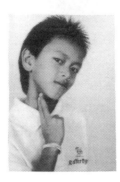

3. Count your pulse for 15 seconds.
   Either have someone else time for you, or watch the second hand on a clock.

4. Multiply your pulse by 4 or use the Heart-Rate Chart to determine the number of pulses or beats per minute.
   Usually, exercising and resting pulses are measured in beats per minute. You don't have to count for 60 seconds to get an accurate reading though.

5. Now, try to find your pulse at your wrist. Place the flat part of two fingers of one hand on the thumb side of your other wrist as shown in Figure 2.9. Feel between the bones and above the wrist joint. Press in lightly.

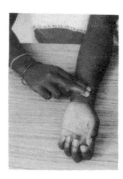

6. Take your pulse a few different times to practice.
   Try taking your pulse at your wrist and at the side of your neck. Do you get a similar pulse rate each time?

7.   With a partner, practice taking one another's pulse.
     You might take your pulse at the side of your neck while your partner takes your pulse at your wrist. Then, compare numbers. Did you get the same number of beats in 15 seconds? If not, practice until you do. Take your partner's pulse in the same way. Remember, your pulse rate will probably not be the same as your partner's pulse rate, but you should be able to agree on each person's pulse rate.

8.   In the next lesson, you need to be able to find your pulse quickly. Practice until you feel you can find your pulse within 2 to 3 seconds.

WRAP UP

Many fitness experts say that

- fitness is for a lifetime,
- fitness is for everyone, and
- fitness should be fun and enjoyable.

Discuss these three concepts. How can you make fitness enjoyable? Why do people need to think about fitness for a lifetime? How can everyone become fit?

Add any ideas to the lists you made in the activity "What Do You Know About Fitness?" Did you learn anything new about physical fitness in this lesson? Did you think of any other benefits of being or becoming physically fit?

INVOLVING FAMILY MEMBERS

Ask your family members what they think about physical fitness. Do they think physical fitness is important? If they are not very active, ask them why they do not exercise much. If they are active, ask them to tell you about the benefits they find from physical fitness activities.

Start planning fun activities that you might do together as a family to enjoy the benefits of becoming fit.

LESSON 3

MEASURING FITNESS

Before you begin any exercise or activity program to improve your physical fitness, it is important for you to know your starting point. How fit are you now? How fit would you like to be? The purpose of fitness testing is <u>not</u> to compare your level of fitness with someone else's. The purpose of testing is to give you a starting point from which you can measure your own improvement. Each person is unique and has a different physical make-up and history. Your results are for your own use. You do not need to share them with anyone else, but you need to know where you are now so you can plan what you need to do to become more physically fit.

Be sure you have on comfortable clothes and proper shoes for exercising. Get yourself psyched up for measuring fitness. Ready, set, go for it!

ACTIVITY: HOW FIT ARE YOU?

Procedure

1. Find a partner. Get a pencil and a record page, titled My Results Record Page, from your teacher.
    You will need a partner to complete most of the fitness tasks. Your partner will keep track of the time for each task, count the number of sit-ups or chin-ups, hold your ankles, read the measurement for the sit-and-reach task, and offer general encouragement. Choose a partner with whom you feel comfortable. Each of you will record your results on your own record page.

2. Follow your teacher's directions for completing each fitness task.
    You will complete such fitness tasks as the mile run, bent-knee sit-ups, chin-ups, and a sit-and-reach task. Your teacher will tell you where and when to do the tasks. Warm up before you complete each task.

3. After you complete each task, record the time, number, or distance on My Results Record Page in the appropriate space.
    Complete all of the fitness tasks before going on to Step 4.

4. Look at the tables that follow. In each table, locate the column for your gender (boy or girl) and age. Find your results in that column. On your record page, write the rating—Keep Up the Good Work, Doing OK, or Improvement Is Possible—that corresponds with your results.

5. Complete the first sentence on the record page under the heading, Moving On.
    Select the one area that you would most like to improve. Although you might want to improve in all areas, pick the one that is most important to you right now. You will be more likely to be successful if you don't try to fix everything all at once.

Rating Tables for Fitness Task Results

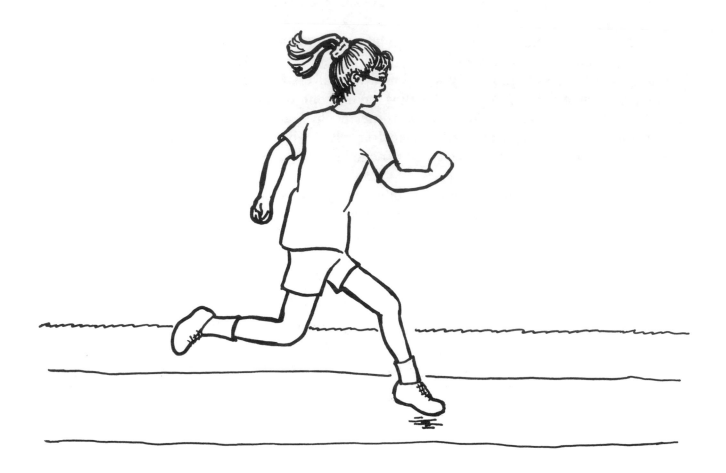

MILE RUN CHART (IN MINUTES AND SECONDS)

Rating	BOYS (BY AGE)					GIRLS (BY AGE)				
	10	11	12	13	14	10	11	12	13	14
Keep up the good work	Less than 9:02	Less than 8:12	Less than 8:03	Less than 7:24	Less than 7:18	Less than 10:27	Less than 10:10	Less than 10:05	Less than 9:48	Less than 9:31
Doing OK	9:02 to 11:00	8:12 to 10:32	8:03 to 10:13	7:24 to 9:10	7:18 to 9:06	10:27 to 12:52	10:10 to 12:54	10:05 to 12:33	9:48 to 12:17	9:31 to 11:49
Improvement is possible	More than 11:00	More than 10:32	More than 10:13	More than 9:10	More than 9:06	More than 12:52	More than 12:54	More than 12:33	More than 12:17	More than 11:49

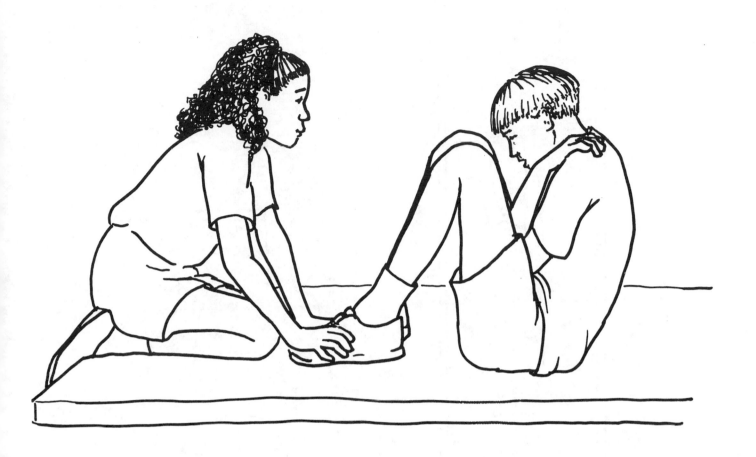

SIT-UPS CHART (NUMBER COMPLETED)

	BOYS (BY AGE)					GIRLS (BY AGE)				
Rating	10	11	12	13	14	10	11	12	13	14
Keep up the good work	More than 38	More than 40	More than 43	More than 45	More than 45	More than 36	More than 36	More than 39	More than 39	More than 40
Doing OK	28 to 38	30 to 40	32 to 43	32 to 45	35 to 45	25 to 36	26 to 36	27 to 39	28 to 39	29 to 40
Improvement is possible	Less than 28	Less than 30	Less than 32	Less than 32	Less than 35	Less than 25	Less than 26	Less than 27	Less than 28	Less than 29

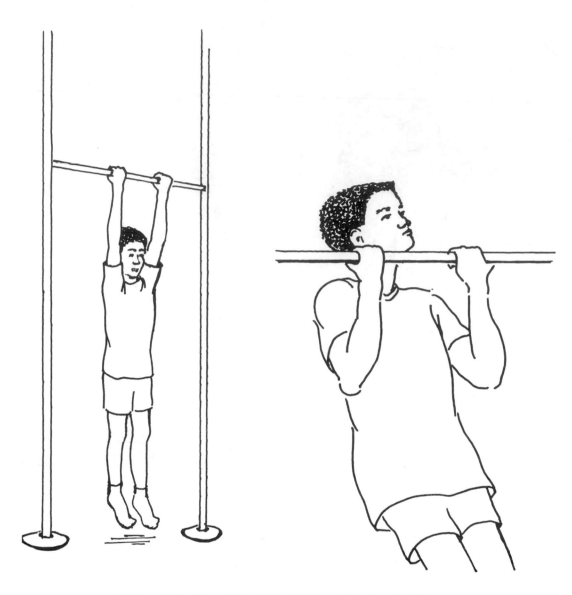

CHIN-UPS CHART (NUMBER COMPLETED)

	BOYS (BY AGE)					GIRLS (BY AGE)				
Rating	10	11	12	13	14	10	11	12	13	14
Keep up the good work	More than 4	More than 4	More than 5	More than 7	More than 8	More than 1	More than 1	More than 1	More than 1	More than 1
Doing OK	1 to 4	1 to 4	1 to 5	1 to 7	2 to 8	1	1	1	1	1
Improvement is possible	Less than 1	Less than 1	Less than 1	Less than 1	Less than 2	Less than 1	Less than 1	Less than 1	Less than 1	Less than 1

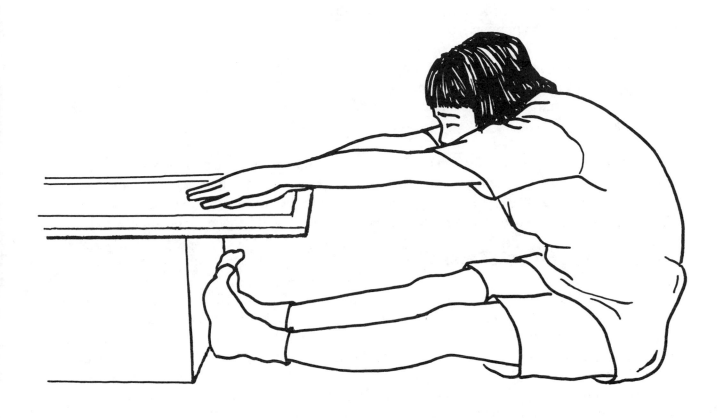

SIT-AND-REACH CHART (IN INCHES)

	BOYS (BY AGE)					GIRLS (BY AGE)				
Rating	10	11	12	13	14	10	11	12	13	14
Keep up the good work	More than 14.5	More than 14.5	More than 14.5	More than 14.5	More than 15.0	More than 16.0	More than 16.5	More than 17.0	More than 17.5	More than 18.0
Doing OK	11.5 to 14.5	11.5 to 14.5	11.0 to 14.5	11.0 to 14.5	11.0 to 15.0	13.0 to 16.0	13.0 to 16.5	14.0 to 17.0	14.0 to 17.5	15.0 to 18.0
Improvement is possible	Less than 11.5	Less than 11.5	Less than 11.0	Less than 11.0	Less than 11.0	Less than 13.0	Less than 13.0	Less than 14.0	Less than 14.0	Less than 15.0

WRAP UP

With your classmates, brainstorm ways you could improve all areas of fitness. What exercises or activities might you do to get your chin over the chin-up bar more times? What might get you in shape to run the mile in less time? How often do you think you might need to do these exercises or activities? Over what period of time?

Use the results from your brainstorming session and complete the second sentence on your record page: I can improve my performance by _____. You can list many ways to improve your performance in the area you chose, but write only those activities or exercises that you are likely to do.

Don't be discouraged if you are disappointed with your results. Most of us would like to be more physically fit, but you can only start from where you are. Now, you have the chance to work hard so that you will do better next time. Just like most things that are worth having, physical fitness takes time and perseverance. It won't happen overnight, but it <u>will</u> happen if you stick with it.

INVOLVING FAMILY MEMBERS

Measure the levels of fitness of your family members. Have family members complete the same fitness tasks you did in class. Make sure everyone warms up ahead of time and does not overdo it. (Do not have very young brothers and sisters do exactly the same tasks. They should not try to run a mile, for example, and they might not be able to do chin-ups or sit-ups. You can think up simple tasks for them to do, such as running back and forth between two chairs a few times, and using their arms to push themselves up from the floor.) Choose one or two areas of fitness to work on as a family. Plan some fun activities you could do a few times a week that would improve your fitness, too.

LESSON 4

WORKING OUT

ACTIVITY: COUNT THE BEATS

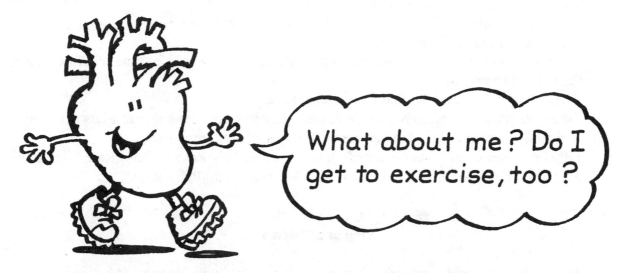

What about me? Do I get to exercise, too?

Every time your heart muscles squeeze or contract, your heart pumps blood throughout your body. Blood travels through the blood vessels to all parts of the body. Arteries carry blood from the heart through the body, and veins carry the blood from the body back to the heart.

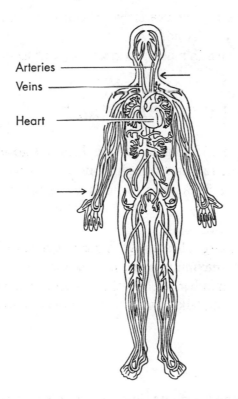

Do the muscles of your heart exercise when you do? Do the following experiment and find out whether your heart muscles exercise when you exercise.

27

Procedure

1. Take out a sheet of paper and a pencil. Sit quietly for 2 or 3 minutes. Locate your pulse at either your neck or your wrist.
2. When your teacher gives a signal to start, count the number of times you feel a beat. Stop counting when your teacher tells you to stop.
3. Write the number of beats you counted.
   Multiply the number by 4 or use the Heart-Rate Chart (if the teacher used a 15-second count) and compute beats per minute.
4. Discuss with your classmates whether a person's pulse rate would be faster or slower when the heart is exercising.
5. Participate in the exercises that your teacher leads.
6. Take your pulse immediately after exercising and compute the number of beats per minute. Write this number next to the number of beats per minute from Step 3.
7. Label the number of beats per minute from Step 3 as "My Resting Pulse Rate." Label the number of beats per minute from Step 6 as "My Exercising Pulse Rate."

Stop and Discuss

1. Was your pulse rate higher or lower after exercising? How much higher or lower?
2. Do you think your heart muscles exercised when you did? What is your evidence?
3. Do you think it is a good idea for your heart to exercise along with your other muscles? Why or why not?
4. What part of fitness is most important for your heart?

ACTIVITY: FINDING MY TARGET HEART RATE

During aerobic exercises, if your pulse rate does not go up enough, your heart will not become more fit. If your pulse rate is too high, your heart is working too hard. That could be dangerous. The ideal pulse rate for a person who is doing aerobic exercises is called the **target heart rate**.

You can calculate your target heart rate. Your target heart rate is really a target heart-rate zone with 70 percent of your maximum heart rate as the low number and 85 percent of your maximum heart rate as the high number. Follow the procedures and calculate your target heart-rate zone. (If you have a heart problem, talk to your doctor. Find out how much you can safely exercise your heart.)

Procedure

1. First, find your maximum heart rate (in beats per minute) by subtracting your age from the number 220. Write that number at the top of a sheet of paper.

For example, Monique is 13 years old. Her maximum heart rate is 220 - 13 = 207 beats per minute. That is as fast as her heart can beat. She should not make her heart work that hard for very long.

2. Multiply your maximum heart rate from Step 1 by 70 percent. Write that number at the left side of your paper.

   That number is the low side of your target heart-rate zone. In Monique's example, her low number will be 70 percent of 207 (207 X .70 = 144.9), which can be rounded off to 145 beats per minute.

3. Next, multiply your maximum heart rate from Step 1 by 85 percent. Write that number at the right side of your paper.

   That number is the high side of your target heart-rate zone. In Monique's example, her high number will be 85 percent of 207 (207 X .85 = 175.9), which can be rounded off to 176 beats per minute.

4. Divide the two numbers of your target heart-rate zone by 4 to find the number of beats you should count in 15 seconds if you are in your zone. (Or, you can use the Heart-Rate Chart. Remember, 15 seconds is one-fourth of one minute.)

   Monique would divide 145 and 176 beats per minute by 4 to get the number of beats in 15 seconds. (145 ÷ 4 = 36; 176 ÷ 4 = 44) This means she should count somewhere between 36 and 44 beats in 15 seconds if she is in her zone.

5. After you have calculated your target heart-rate zone and know the number of beats you should count in 15 seconds, try some aerobic exercises, such as running in place or jumping jacks, for a minute or two. Take your pulse for 15 seconds after exercising and find out if you are in your zone.

   If your heart beats more times that your high number, you are working too hard and you should slow down. If your heart beats fewer times than your low number, you are not working hard enough and should try to speed up a little.

6. Practice as you exercise. Stop and check your pulse rate once in a while during aerobic exercise. Count the beats for only 15 seconds to avoid stopping for very long. Are you exercising within your zone?

READING: WHAT IS "WORKING OUT"?

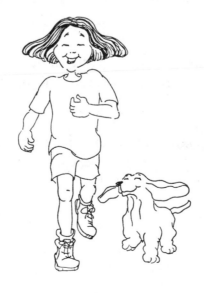

What does "working out" mean to you? You might think of athletes in training. They "work out" to stay in condition for their sport. You might think of people lifting weights in a gym. They "work out" to become stronger and to stay in shape. You might think of certain actresses and actors who advertise their own "workout" programs. They sell books and videotapes to convince other people to exercise along with them. Are there other ways to "work out"? Does a workout always have to be "work"? Did you know that you can work out without being an athlete and without a gym or a videotape?

In this lesson, you will experience a lot of the information you have learned so far in this unit. In the second lesson, you read and talked about fitness and all the areas of physical fitness. In the third lesson, you tested your level of fitness in different areas and set goals for personal improvement. Now, in this lesson, you can put all those lessons to work. You will participate in a complete physical fitness "workout" that will help you learn about warming up and cooling down, what cardiovascular or aerobic activity really feels like—be prepared to breathe hard and to feel your heart beat faster!—and what types of exercises will improve your muscle tone.

Your teacher will lead you through a complete workout that will go something like this:

You will do some slow stretching and moving exercises for about 5 minutes to warm up your muscles (including your heart) to get ready for faster activity.

Next, you will participate in some fast activities for about 15 or 20 minutes, maybe aerobic dancing or basketball or running games. This is the aerobic part of the workout that works your heart and lungs and gets a lot of oxygen moving through your blood to all parts of your body. You can practice taking your heart rate during this part of the workout. Always try to exercise hard enough to stay within your zone but not above it. You won't help your heart and will just get tired if you work above your zone.

Next, for about 10 minutes, you will complete some exercises that will make the muscles in your legs, arms, stomach, chest, and back stronger and able to work longer.

Finally, for the last 5 minutes, you will stretch out the muscles that you've been working so hard so that you feel relaxed and refreshed and not tired after working out.

That's what we call "working out." It does take some work, but it's really more fun than work. After you try working out three times a week for a few weeks in a row, review your list of the benefits of physical activity from Lesson 2. How many have you experienced? Are you feeling good and looking good?

ACTIVITY: IT'S TIME TO WORK OUT!

As you participate in a complete workout with your teacher and classmates, pay attention to how you feel during the parts of the workout. Is your heart beating fast? Does your breathing rate increase? Work at your own pace and enjoy your fitness experience.

WRAP UP

Relate the parts of the workout to the components of fitness. Which parts of the workout will improve your cardiovascular fitness, your strength, your endurance, your flexibility? Why are all parts of the workout necessary for overall fitness?

Talk about your reaction to "working out." Did you enjoy the workout? Which parts did you like best? What would you like to do more of? Less of? How would you like to change the workout next time?

Share your thoughts with your teacher and classmates. Discuss how to make the workouts fun for everyone.

INVOLVING FAMILY MEMBERS

Lead your family in a workout. Before you begin, have each member take a pulse rate and find beats per minute. Then, as you work out, take pulse rates right after the cardiovascular section and again after the "cool down." Compare the pulse rates of members of the family. Were younger members' pulse rates lower or higher than the older people's? Why do you think the pulse rates were different for different people?

If you have "workout videos" at home, evaluate those workout plans. Do they provide for all components of fitness? Do they start with a warm-up that lasts at least 5 minutes? Do they end with a cool-down that stretches the muscles? Use video workouts only if they include all components of fitness.

LESSON 5

S-T-R-E-T-C-H IT!

Stretching is one of the best ways to improve and maintain flexibility. Stretching feels good when you do it correctly. You do not have to push yourself and try to go farther each day. Stretching should be something personal, not a competition to see who can stretch farther. Some people have more flexible joints and muscles than others, so you could hurt your muscles and joints if you try to stretch farther than your joints or muscles will allow.

Stretching meets the needs of your body. It is a painless way to get your body ready for movement. When you stretch regularly and correctly, you can avoid injuries and perform to the best of your ability.

Remember to take it slowly, especially at the beginning. Start easy, but stretch often. When you take time to stretch out your muscles and limber up your joints, you will enjoy your activities even more.

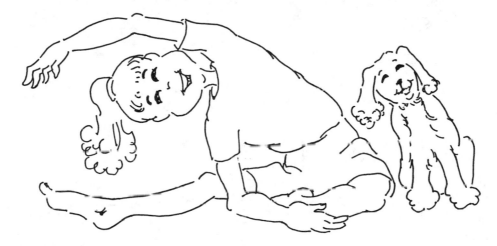

ACTIVITY: STRETCHING OUT

Procedure

1. Stand up and move about a little. Think about how tense or relaxed your body feels and make a mental note about how you feel.
    For example, where would you place yourself on a "tenseness" scale of 1 to 10?

Very tense				*A Little Tense*				*Relaxed*	
1	*2*	*3*	*4*	*5*	*6*	*7*	*8*	*9*	*10*

2   Perform the stretches described below.
    Be sure to wear comfortable, loose-fitting clothes. Stretch only as far as your joints and muscles will allow. Don't bounce while you stretch; maintain a slow, even stretch.

3. Stand up and move about again. How tense or relaxed does your body feel now?
    Where would you rate yourself now on the "tenseness" scale? Are you more relaxed than before?

1.   Upper Body Stretch

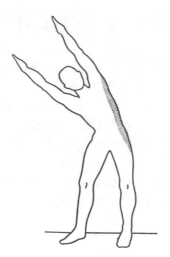

Stand erect, feet about shoulder width apart, arms raised over your head, palms facing each other. Bending at the waist, make a complete rotation of your upper body. Keep knees relaxed, not locked.

2.   The Calf Stretch

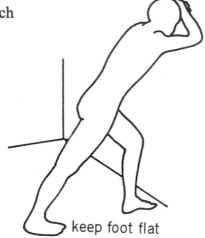

keep foot flat

Face a wall, standing 12 to 15 inches away from it. Lean against the wall, resting your forearms on the wall and your forehead on the backs of your hands. Bend one knee, moving that foot toward the wall. The back leg should be straight with the foot flat (heel down) and pointed straight ahead. Slowly move your hips forward, still keeping the back leg straight and foot flat. Create an easy stretch in your calf muscle and hold for 20 to 30 seconds. Now stretch the other calf muscle.

The stretching activities were excerpted from *STRETCHING*© 1980 by Bob & Jean Anderson. Shelter Publications, Bolinas, CA. Distributed in bookstores by Random House. Reprinted by permission. For a free catalog of Stretching Inc. products/publications contact: Stretching, Inc., P. O. Box 767, Palmer Lake, CO 80133 or call 800-333-1307.

3.   Hamstring Stretch #1

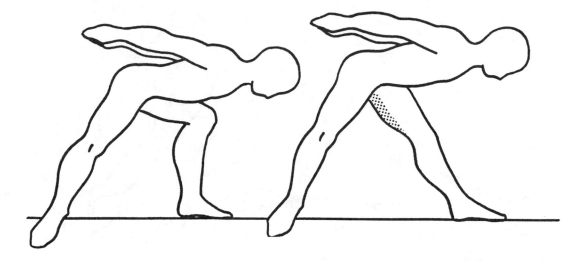

Stand in straddle position (facing forward with feet six to eight inches apart) with toes pointing forward. Turn left foot to the left and bend the left knee, keeping your body weight over the left leg. Keep right leg straight with right foot facing forward. Place hands behind back. Bend so that the chest is parallel to the floor. While holding that position, slowly straighten the left leg and hold for 15 to 30 seconds. Repeat with right leg. You should feel the stretch in the hamstring.

4.   Hip Flexor Stretch

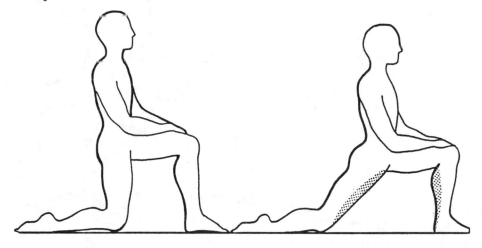

Place right knee on the floor behind left foot. Move left knee forward so that it is positioned over the toes. Place palms on left knee facing toward the floor. Make sure knee and toes are pointing forward and not to the side. Hold for 15 to 30 seconds. Repeat with left leg. The stretch should be felt in front of the hip and possibly in the groin and hamstrings.

5.   Hamstring Stretch #2

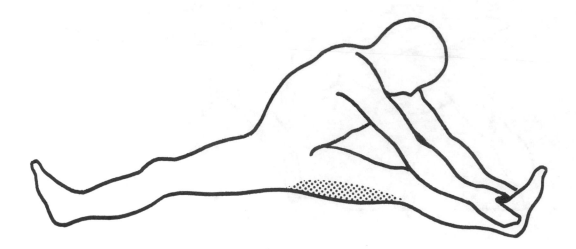

Sit on the floor with both legs out straight and approximately three to four feet apart with ankles flexed (toes straight up). Lean upper body toward the left leg bending at the hips. Keep your lower back flat. Hold for 15 to 30 seconds. Repeat with right leg. You should feel the stretch in the hamstring and lower back.

6.   Gluteal Stretch

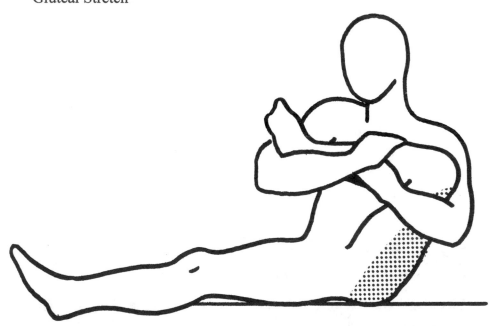

Sit with both legs out in front of you. Slip both arms around left leg and raise leg up and toward chest. Keep lower back flat. Hold for 15 to 20 seconds. Repeat with right leg. You should feel the stretch in the outer thigh and buttocks.

7.　　Groin Stretch

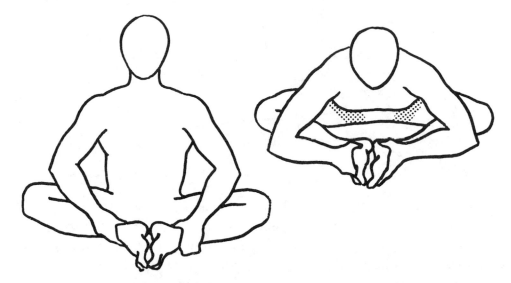

Sit on the floor with the soles of your feet together. Put your hands around your feet so that your elbows are slightly in front of your lower legs. Gently pull your body forward until you feel a stretch in your inner thigh (groin) area. Keep your lower back flat; do not bend your head down toward your hands. Face forward. Increase the stretch until you feel tension but not pain. Hold the stretch for 30 seconds and concentrate on how your muscles feel. Release the stretch slowly.

8.　　Quadricep Stretch

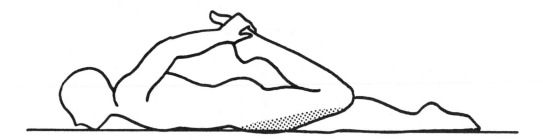

Lie on stomach with head down. With right hand, pull right foot toward the buttocks. Hold for 15 to 30 seconds. Repeat with left leg. You should feel the stretch in the quadricep muscle, the large muscle at the front of the thigh.

9.   Lower Back Stretch

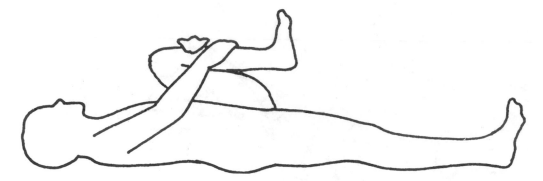

Lie on your back. Bend one knee toward your chest. Grasp your leg just below the knee and gently pull your knee toward your chest. You should feel a stretch in the back of your leg. Keep your lower back pressed into the floor while you stretch. Hole the stretch for 30 seconds. Release slowly and stretch the other leg.

As a variation, stretch the outside of your leg by pulling the bent leg slightly toward the opposite shoulder. Keep your back flat on the floor. Hold for 20 seconds. Do both legs, one at a time.

Stretch both legs by bringing both knees into the chest. First keep your head down, then curl your head up toward your knees and hold that position. Then, straighten out your legs and arms and relax.

10.   Whole Body Stretch

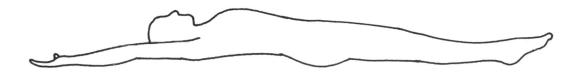

Lie on your back with your arms straight over your head and legs extended straight in front. Stretch arms and legs (point the toes) feeling as though you are making your body longer. Pull in your abdominal muscles to make the middle of your body thin and press the small of your back into the floor. Hold this stretch for five seconds. Release. Repeat the stretch three times. This stretch is good for your arms, shoulders, spine, abdominal muscles, legs, feet, and ankles.

ACTIVITY: WORKING OUT

Now that you have stretched and loosened your muscles and joints, you are ready for some aerobic activity. Join your classmates and teacher in today's fitness fun.

WRAP UP

Find books or magazine articles on fitness at the library. What do the experts say about stretching as a part of overall fitness? Take notes on the recommendations you find about how to stretch properly and prepare to explain or demonstrate some of those procedures for the class.

INVOLVING FAMILY MEMBERS

Introduce your family to stretching. Lead a stretching session at home and ask your family members to think about how tense their bodies feel before and after stretching. You might hold a stretching session during a television show and lead a different stretch or two during each commercial break.

BECOMING STRONGER

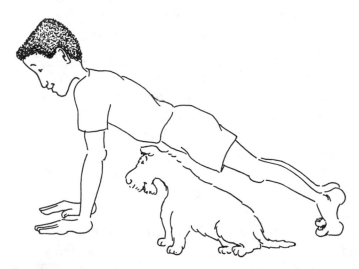

All of us need well-toned, well-defined muscles that allow us to move easily, to participate in daily activities without tiring, to walk and sit with good posture, and to look our best. How can we keep our muscles toned and strong? — not by sitting around watching MTV. That's for sure! Let's get busy...

ACTIVITY: BODY STRENGTH

Procedure

1. Read the exercising tips that follow. Discuss their importance with your teacher and classmates.

Exercising Do's and Don'ts

- Perform conditioning exercises carefully and with control. Rapid repetitions are not safe.
- Do not hold your breath while you exercise. Practice good breathing techniques by exhaling when you are contracting your muscles.
- Use a mat or carpeted surface for floor exercises.
- Make sure you are not arching your back during the exercises. Keep your lower back flat or pressed into the floor or mat at all times.
- Perform repetitions until you feel the muscles fatiguing. Then, do a few more repetitions, but do not push yourself to the point of pain. Pain can mean injury.
- Be sensible when using weights. You should be able to complete a set of 10 to 12 repetitions without stopping. If you are unable to complete 10 repetitions, you are probably using too much weight.

> - Follow these general guidelines:
>
>   Beginner -- 1 set of 10 to 12 repetitions
>
>   Intermediate-- 2 sets of 10 to 12 repetitions
>
>   Advanced -- 3 sets of 10 to 12 repetitions
>
> Work up from one level to the next. Do not assume you are ready for the advanced stage until you have successfully completed the other two.

2. Warm up by completing some of the stretches from Lesson 5.
   Choose stretches that will relax and stretch out all parts of your body--your legs, your arms, your back, your shoulders, and your abdomen.

3. Perform the exercises for muscular strength that follow.
   If you have not exercised much lately, your muscles will be out of shape. Start easy and remember that this is not a competition to see who can do more repetitions. When you become tired or your muscles feel sore, stop. You can injure your muscles or joints if you work them too hard before you are ready.

4. Stretch out the muscles that you worked during this session.

5. Make a note of which exercises were easy for you to do and which were difficult.
   You should spend more time with the exercises that were difficult, gradually increasing the number of repetitions.

6. Read the information that follows about specificity and overload.
   The information should help you decide which muscles to work on and how to make them stronger without injury.

Exercises for Muscular Strength

Exercises for Strong Abdominal (Stomach) Muscles   (from easy to more difficult)

1. Pelvic Tilt

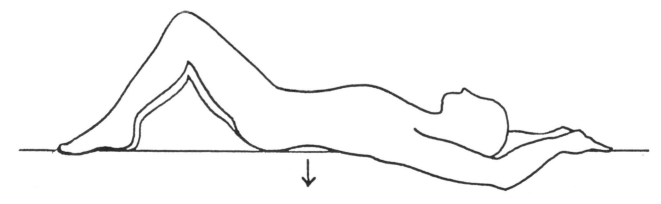

Lie on your back with your knees bent and feet flat on the floor, slightly apart. Press the lower part of your back down to the floor by contracting your abdominal and gluteal (buttocks) muscles. Hold the contraction for about five seconds. The lumbar spine (lower portion of the spine) should be pressed firmly against the mat or floor. Release and repeat.

2.   Upper Abdominal Curls

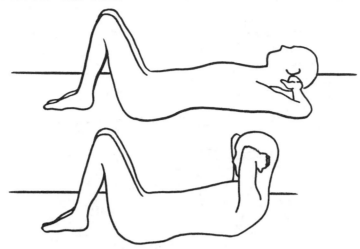

Lie on your back with your knees bent. Place your fingertips behind your head, just slightly behind your ears. (Do not place your hands all the way behind your head because you might pull up too hard on your neck.) Focus your eyes toward the ceiling and hold your chin away from your chest. Relax your neck and shoulders. Curl upper body forward and up until your shoulders lift from the floor. Tighten your upper abdominal muscles as you curl up. Hold for 5 seconds and then repeat.

3.   Lower Abdominal Curls

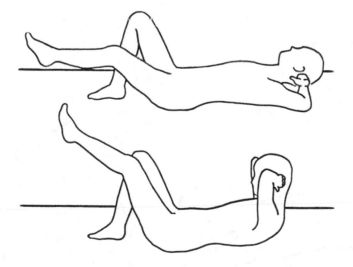

Lie on your back with one leg outstretched and opposite knee bent. Place hands behind head, as in Upper Abdominal Curls, with fingertips just behind ears. Together, curl the torso forward as you lift the extended leg no higher than the top of the bent knee. Be sure to tighten your abdominal muscles to pull yourself up and do not pull on your neck. Repeat same movement raising other leg.

4.   Abdominal Obliques

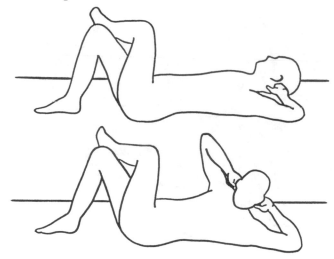

Lie on back with right leg bent and opposite leg crossed over the knee. Place hands behind head with fingertips just behind ears. Slowly twist the torso bringing the right shoulder toward the left knee of the crossed leg. Do not pull on your head neck to lift yourself; use your abdominal muscles. Repeat the same movement on the other side.

5.   Advanced Upper Abdominal Curls

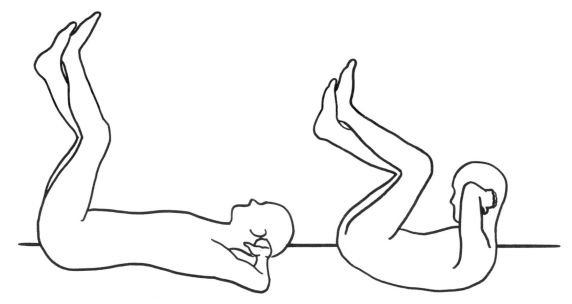

Lie on your back with your legs elevated into the air and ankles crossed. Hold hands behind head with fingertips just behind ears. Keep your lower back pressed into the floor. Draw your knees toward your chest as you curl your upper body forward.

1.   Leg Lifts

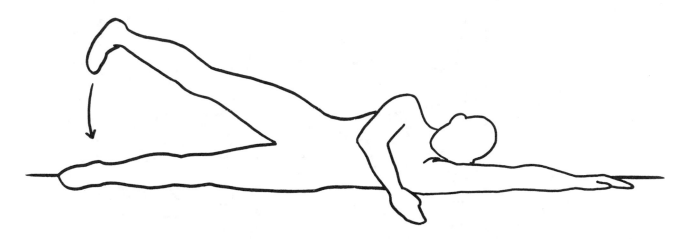

Lie on one side with head resting on shoulder, lower arm extended.
Lift top leg to about a 45 degree angle and gradually lower it. (Lower
leg can be bent or straight.) Muscles get the best workout when toes
of upper leg are turned downward to that toes touch heel of lower foot
when leg is lowered. Move leg slowly up and down; don't let gravity
take over on way down, but control the downward movement.
Repeat with other leg.

2.   Cross Leg Lifts

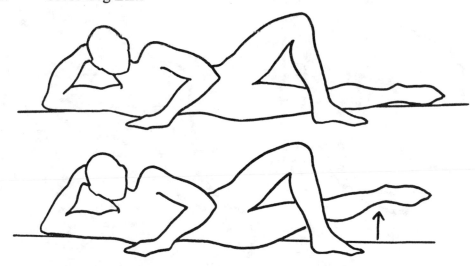

Lie on one side with legs straight. Prop yourself up on your elbow
with head resting on hand, other arm in front, palm on floor for
balance. Bend your top leg and place that foot on the floor just in
front of your bottom knee. While in that position, raise and lower
your bottom leg. Switch sides.

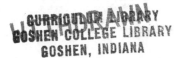

3.   Reverse Leg Lift

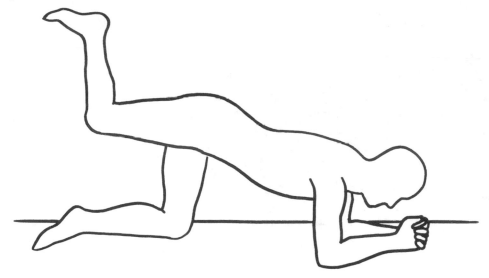

Balance on knees and forearms with hands clasped in front. Slightly round back and keep head low. Lift one leg, bend at the knee, and flex foot. Press sole of foot toward ceiling until knee lines up with buttocks. (Thigh will be parallel to floor.) Lower leg a few inches. Continue to press sole of foot toward ceiling and lower in gentle up and down motion. Tighten the buttocks as you press toward ceiling. Repeat with other leg.

4.   Doggie

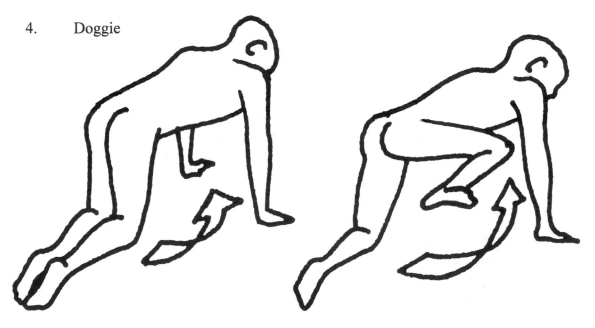

Balance on hands and knees keeping head straight forward and back level or slightly rounded. (Do not let back arch.) Lift right leg to side with knee bent. Leg forms a right angle to body when lifted. Lower leg and repeat. Repeat with other leg. Be sure body stays straight; do not rock or lean to the side. Tighten buttocks as you lift leg.

5.   Wall Sit

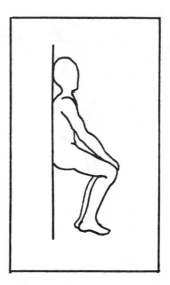

Stand with your back flat against a wall. Move your feet out about 12 inches from the wall as you lower yourself to a sitting position so that your legs form a right angle at the knees. (Your thighs should be parallel to the floor.) You should feel as though you are sitting in an imaginary chair. Hold that position as long as you can. Stand up and relax. Lower yourself again and hold. Repeat as many times as possible.

Exercises for Strong Arms and Upper Body (from easy to more difficult)

1.   Wall Push-ups

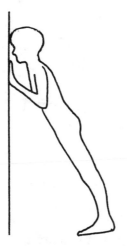 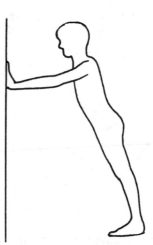

Stand facing the wall with feet about 15 inches from the wall. Lean against the wall with palms flat against the wall, elbows bent, nose to wall. Hands should be about shoulder level. Push body away from wall until arms are fully extended. Bend arms to return nose to wall. Push away again. Repeat.

2.　　Extended Arm Circles

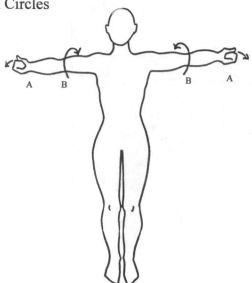

In standing position, hold arms straight out at shoulder level, palms facing ceiling. Make fists and move arms in small circles going forward. Change directions and make circles going backward. Gradually make circles larger and rotate through shoulder joint. Gradually make circles smaller again.

3.　　Platter Lift

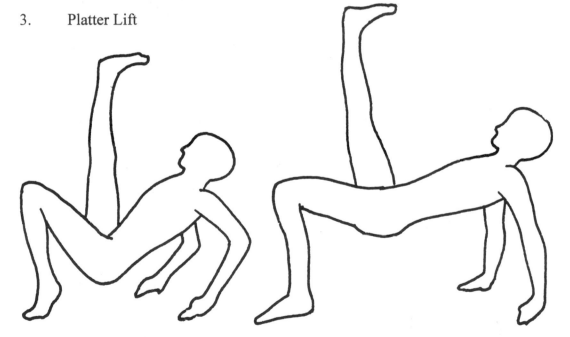

Assume crab position facing toward ceiling. Palms and feet are flat on the floor, knees and elbows are bent. Lift one leg to a vertical position with foot flexed as though you were balancing a platter on the bottom of your foot. Raise and lower body by bending at the elbows keeping your leg straight up the entire time. Raise your hips as high as you can off the floor when you straighten your arms.

4.   Arm Curls

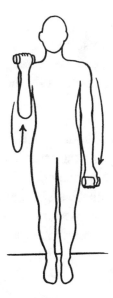

Hold small weights or a soup can in each hand. Hold arms down at sides with palms forward. Bend elbows and bring weights up to shoulders and gradually lower. Do one arm at a time or both arms together. To vary exercise, hold arms straight out in front with palms up, bend elbows, bring weights to shoulders and back out again. Or, hold arms out to sides, shoulder high, with palms up and bring weights to shoulders and back out again.

5.   Push-ups

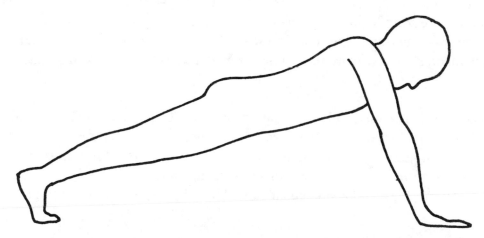

One of the best exercises for increasing upper body strength is the push-up. Lie on your stomach with your hands on either side of your shoulders. (Elbows will be bent.) Push body up with arms until arms are straight. You can use either your toes or knees as the contact point with the floor. (Push-ups from the knees are easier than push-ups from the toes.) Lower body so that nose nearly touches the floor; do not let chest touch the floor. As you raise and lower body, keep body in a straight line with back flat.

READING: SPECIFICITY AND OVERLOAD

To be physically fit, you need strong muscles. Those muscles don't have to be as strong as a body builder's muscles, they just have to be strong enough to allow you to move easily in all directions without injuring yourself. Muscular strength and endurance are part of the important components of overall fitness.

There are two ideas about strengthening your muscles that you should understand before you begin an exercise program. One is **specificity** and the other is **overload**. Specificity is pretty simple. It means that only specific exercises will strengthen specific muscles. In other words, abdominal curls or crunches will make your stomach muscles stronger, but they won't do a thing for your thighs. Chin-ups or push-ups will make your arms stronger, but they still won't get at those thighs. You have to do the specific exercises that make particular muscles stronger. If you want to improve your performance on the chin-ups task, for example, then you must perform exercises that use and strengthen the muscles in your upper body.

Overload is a bit harder to figure out because it will be different for each person. Basically, overload means that your muscles will not become stronger unless you exercise them at a higher-than-normal level. You have to push your muscles a little beyond what they can already do. Once your muscles are stronger through exercise, the exercises will become easier and you can move from the beginner to the intermediate level. The secret is to know your own body and to work at a level that is best for you.

In developing muscular strength and endurance, concentrate mainly on three muscle groups: the abdominal (stomach) muscles, the muscles of the legs and buttocks, and the muscles of the upper body (arms, chest, and shoulders). Notice that the exercises you performed in this lesson were divided into those three specific groups. Usually, some muscle groups are stronger than others. This will vary from person to person. You should work all three muscle groups, but especially those that are weak. Remember, start easy with weak muscles. You must strengthen them gradually over time to avoid injury.

If you are worried about developing bulging muscles, doing exercises for muscular strength and endurance won't make you look like Arnold Schwarzenegger. You must go through very specialized training programs to build big muscles like his. Exercises for muscular strength will make your muscles stronger, keep your skin looking healthier and less baggy, and will give definition to your arms, legs, and abdomen. You will look better, not muscle-bound.

Stop and Discuss

1. Describe exercises that are specific to the upper body, the abdomen, and the legs and buttocks. Explain the principle of specificity as it relates to those exercises.
2. How will you know if you are applying the principle of overload appropriately?
3. What are the benefits of developing muscular strength and endurance?
4. How might you improve muscular strength and endurance during daily activities?

WRAP UP

Work with a partner or in a team and design a poster that shows what strong muscles can do for you. Think about the benefits of having strong muscles. Will you look better? Will you feel better? Will you be able to leap tall buildings in a single bound?

Write a message on the poster that will encourage you and others to become stronger.

INVOLVING FAMILY MEMBERS

Develop a circuit training course at home. Find a good place for abdominal exercises, another for arm and upper body conditioning, and a third for leg exercises. Post signs at each training location. Teach your family members the proper way to do each exercise. Then, complete the circuit every other day. Keep track of how each person feels at the end of each week. Do they find daily activities easier to perform as they become stronger?

THE FITNESS-NUTRITION CONNECTION

An important part of fitness is maintaining a lean body. A lean body is not necessarily a small body. A lean body has enough fat for warmth, for protection, and for padding, but does not have extra fat. Acquiring a lean body can involve gaining or losing fat, which is your body's storage of energy. Look at the following equations for a general idea of how to maintain a lean body.

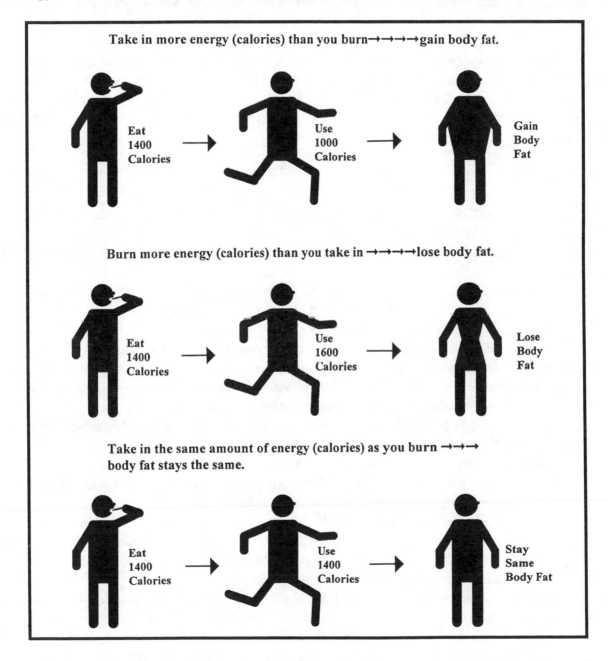

This gives you a general picture of the fitness-nutrition connection, but how do you know if you are in balance? The next activity will give you some ideas.

ACTIVITY: BALANCING ENERGY NEEDS

Teenagers need about 2,400 calories a day. (The number of calories each teenager needs varies, but you can use 2,400 calories for the purposes of this activity.) What are calories anyway? Calories are a measure of the amount of energy in food. The typical teenager needs about 2,400 calories worth of energy from food to grow, to move, and to stay healthy. A food's energy comes from the sugars, starches, fats, and proteins that it contains. Some people think vitamins give them energy, but vitamins have no calories. (Although vitamins do not give you energy, they do help you use the energy in foods. You need vitamins, minerals, and water, as well as energy, for your body to work properly.)

Because you use more energy when you are active than when you sit around, you might use more than 2,400 calories in a day if you are very active. If you do not get enough energy from the foods you eat, your body gets the energy from the fat stored in your body. If you eat food that provides more energy (calories) than you use, your body stores the extra energy as fat. You need to find the balance that is right for you.

Procedure

1. Look at the Activity Chart that follows the procedures. Choose activities that you would do in <u>one day</u>. Write a list of your choices on a sheet of paper.
2. Next to each activity, write the approximate number of minutes you would do each activity in one day.
3. Calculate the number of calories you would burn if you did each activity for the number of minutes you chose. Write the number of calories next to the activity.
   Choose the weight column that is closest to your weight.
4. Next, write the number of calories you need to grow, move, and stay alive.
   Hint: Read the introduction to the activity for a number that applies to most teenagers.
5. Add the numbers from Steps 3 and 4. Write the total number of calories you would need in a day to do those activities and maintain your body's normal functions.
6. Look at the Food Chart at the end of the lesson. Choose the foods that you would eat in one day. Write your choices on your paper.
   Choose many different foods, enough for a full day's meals. Choose healthy foods--those low in fat and sugar when possible, but choose foods that you would be willing to eat. If a food you like to eat is not on the chart, choose a food that is similar to the food you like.
7. Next to the name of each food, write the number of calories the food provides.
   You might have to multiply or divide the number of calories if you choose a different serving size. An estimate will work for the purposes of this activity.
8. Add the number of calories contained in all the foods you chose.
9. Compare the number of calories you would need for your activities (from Step 5) with the number of calories in all the foods you chose (from Step 8). Which number is larger? To make the numbers the same, would you need to have more or less energy from food?
10. Add or subtract foods from your list (from Step 6) or add activities until the number of calories provided by the foods equals the number of calories you need in a day.
    Notice that if you choose low-calorie foods, you can eat more food.

11. Plan how you would divide the foods during the day. Write "B" next to those foods you would eat for breakfast, "L" next to lunch foods, "D" next to dinner foods, and "S" next to snack foods.

Use each item on your list for only one meal. If you want to eat the same food for two meals, write that food and its number of calories twice.

12. Check your lists again. Make sure you have a balance between the calories you need for your daily activities and the calories you take in from the food you eat. Be prepared to share your lists with the class.

ACTIVITY CHART
Calories Used Per Minute According to Your Weight

	Weight in Pounds		
	100	120	150
Badminton	4.3	5.2	6.5
Bicycling (slow)	3.1	3.8	4.7
Bicycling (moderate)	5.4	6.5	8.1
Calisthenics (exercises)	3.3	3.9	4.9
Cleaning Windows	2.7	3.3	3.8
Conversing	1.2	1.3	1.6
Dancing, vigorous	7.8	9.1	10.0
Dressing or Showering	2.1	2.6	3.2
Eating	1.1	1.3	1.5
Golf	3.6	4.3	5.4
Handball	6.3	7.6	9.5
Housework	2.7	3.1	4.0
Jogging, 11-min. mile	6.1	7.3	9.1
Mountain Climbing	6.6	8.0	10.0
Mowing the Grass	3.2	3.7	4.5
Running, 8-min. mile	9.4	11.3	14.1
Racquetball	6.3	7.6	9.5
School Work	1.2	1.4	1.6
Shoveling Snow	7.9	8.5	10.2

Skating, moderate	3.6	4.3	5.4
Skiing, downhill	6.3	7.6	9.5
Skiing, cross-country	7.2	8.7	10.8
Soccer	6.3	7.6	9.5
Sweeping the Floor	2.4	2.9	3.7
Swimming, crawl stroke	5.8	6.9	8.7
Swimming, breast stroke	4.8	5.7	7.2
Table Tennis	2.7	3.2	4.0
Tennis	4.5	5.4	6.8
Volleyball, moderate	2.3	2.7	3.4
Walking, slow	2.7	3.2	4.0
Walking, moderate	3.9	4.6	5.8
Watching TV	0.9	1.1	1.3

Stop and Discuss

1. Did this activity represent "real life" for you? Why or why not?
2. Which do you think would affect your level of body fat more—dieting or being more active? Give reasons for your answer.
3. Is it healthy to go on diets to maintain your weight? Why or why not?
4. Should you try your best to look like the models on television or in magazines? Why or why not?

WRAP UP

Record everything you eat and drink for two days. (List both what you eat and drink and the amount. If you are not sure of the exact amount, estimate.) Bring your record to class. Use the Food Chart to find out the number of calories you ate in two days. (If a food you ate is not on the Food Chart, then find a food that is similar.) How does the number of calories you actually ate compare to the number of calories you calculated during the activity "Balancing Energy Needs"? Do you think you are eating enough calories for your level of activity? Are you active enough to burn any extra calories you consume? How could you reach a balance?

INVOLVING FAMILY MEMBERS

Make an agreement with family members to try to eat mainly low-fat, low-sugar foods for one week. Make a list of healthy snacks that you could have around the house, such as popcorn (no butter), carrot sticks, fruits, yogurt and frozen yogurt, crackers, smoothies made with low-fat milk and fruit, and chocolate shakes made with low-fat chocolate milk and frozen yogurt. After one week of healthy eating, ask everyone how they feel. Do they feel better and have more energy? If you add healthy eating to regular exercise, you should really feel great!

FOOD CHART

Sugar and fat notes: "Fatty" means the food has a lot of fat. "Some fat" means the food has a medium amount of fat. "Low fat" means the food has a little fat. "Sugary" means the food has a lot of sugar. "Some sugar" means the food has a medium amount of sugar. "Low sugar" means the food has a little sugar, often natural sugar such as that in fruits. If there is no note about sugar or fat, the food has little or no fat or sugar.

Food	Number of Calories in 1 Serving
Dairy Products:	
Milk (whole)	160 calories in 1 cup (fatty)
Milk (skim)	90 calories in 1 cup (low fat)
Chocolate milk (2%)	190 calories in 1 cup (some fat)
Cottage cheese	260 calories in 1 cup (low fat)
Ice cream	95 calories in 1 scoop (3 oz.) (fatty)
Butter pecan ice cream	320 calories in 4 ounces (fatty)
Chocolate ice cream	280 calories in 4 ounces (fatty)
Strawberry ice cream	260 calories in 4 ounces (fatty)
Vanilla ice cream	280 calories in 4 ounces (fatty)
Plain yogurt	125 calories in 1 cup (low fat)
Cream cheese	120 calories in 1 ounce (fatty)
Cheddar cheese	115 calories in 1 ounce (fatty)
American cheese	105 calories in 1 cup (low fat)
Mozzarella cheese	95 calories in 1 ounce (low fat)
Parmesan cheese	100 calories in 1 ounce (fatty)
Swiss cheese	110 calories in 1 ounce (fatty)
Meats & Eggs:	
Egg (boiled)	85 calories in 1 large (cholesterol)
Bacon	90 calories in two slices (fatty)
Pot roast of beef	254 calories in 3 ounces (some fat)
Corned beef	350 calories 4 ounces (some fat)

Steak	330 calories in 3 ounces (some fat)]
Beef stew	210 calories in 1 cup (some fat)
Chili (with beans)	335 calories in 1 cup (some fat)
Roast lamb	235 calories in 3 ounces (some fat)
Ham	245 calories in 3 ounces (some fat)
Ham (canned)	140 calories 4 ounces (fatty)
Pepperoni	270 calories 2 ounces (fatty)
Pork chop	260 calories in 1 thick chop (some fat)
Bologna	80 calories in 2 slices (fatty)
Hamburger (just the meat)	245 calories in 1 patty (fatty)
Hot dog	170 calories in 1 (fatty)
Fried chicken drumstick	90 calories in 1 (some fat)
Fried chicken breast	155 calories in 1 (some fat)
Turkey (roasted)	135 calories 4 ounces (some fat)
Chicken (roasted)	190 calories 4 ounces (some fat)
Flounder (baked)	220 calories in 4 ounces (low fat)
Haddock (broiled)	150 calories 4 ounces (low fat)
Halibut (broiled)	200 calories 4 ounces (low fat)
Salmon (steamed)	225 calories 4 ounces (low fat)
Tuna (fresh, raw)	155 calories 4 ounces (low fat)
Tuna (canned, in water)	120 calories in 4 ounces (low fat)
Tuna (canned, in oil)	500 calories 4 ounces (fatty)
Fish sticks	80 calories in 2 (some fat)
Crabmeat	85 calories in 3 ounces (low fat)
Shrimp	100 calories in 3 ounces (low fat)
Beans & Peanuts:	
Beans (pinto, navy, cooked)	200 calories in 1 cup (low fat)
Peanuts	840 calories in 1 cup (fatty)
Peanut butter	95 calories in 1 tablespoon (fatty)

Vegetables:	
Asparagus	10 calories in 4 pieces
Lima beans	95 calories in 1/2 cup
Green beans	15 calories in 1/2 cup
Bean sprouts	18 calories in 1/2 cup
Beets	30 calories in 1/2 cup
Broccoli	20 calories in 1/2 cup
Brussels sprouts	28 calories in 1/2 cup
Cabbage (cooked)	15 calories in 1/2 cup
Carrot	20 calories in 1 medium
Cauliflower	13 calories in 1/2 cup
Celery	5 calories in 1 stalk
Collards	27 calories in 1/2 cup
Corn	70 calories in 1 ear
Cucumber	30 calories in 1 medium
Lettuce	10 calories in 2 large leaves
Peas	58 calories in 1/2 cup
Baked potato (plain)	90 calories in 1 medium
French fries	150 calories in 10 fries (some fat)
Mashed potatoes	65 calories in 1/2 cup
Potato chips	115 calories in 10 chips (fatty)
Sauerkraut	22 calories in 1/2 cup
Spinach	20 calories in 1/2 cup
Zucchini	15 calories in 1/2 cup
Sweet potato	155 calories in 1 medium
Sweet potato (candied)	295 calories in 1 medium (some sugar)
Tomato	40 calories in 1 medium
Tofu	80 calories (low fat)

Fruits:	
Apple	70 calories in 1 medium
Apple juice	120 calories in 1 cup (some sugar)
Applesauce (sweetened)	230 calories in 1 cup (some sugar)
Banana	100 calories in 1 medium (low sugar)
Blueberries	85 calories in 1 cup (low sugar)
Cantaloupe	60 calories in 1/2 medium (low sugar)
Fruit cocktail	195 calories in 1 cup (some sugar)
Cranapple juice	175 calories 1 cup (some sugar)
Grapefruit	45 calories in 1/2 medium (low sugar)
Grapefruit juice (unsweetened)	90 calories in 1 cup
Grapes	95 calories in 1 cup (low sugar)
Grape juice	135 calories in 1 cup (some sugar)
Lemonade	110 calories in 1 cup (some sugar)
Peach	35 calories in 1 medium (low sugar)
Pear	100 calories in 1 medium (low sugar)
Pineapple (raw)	75 calories in 1 cup (low sugar)
Pineapple (canned, with syrup)	195 calories in 1 cup (some sugar)
Plum	25 calories (low sugar)
Raisins	240 calories in 1/2 cup (sugary)
Strawberries	55 calories in 1 cup (low sugar)
Watermelon	115 calories in 1 wedge (some sugar)
Pasta, Cereals & Baked Goods:	
Macaroni	190 calories in 1 cup
Macaroni and cheese	430 calories in 1 cup (fatty)
Noodles (cooked)	200 calories in 1 cup
Rice (cooked)	110 calories in 1/2 cup
Spaghetti (cooked)	155 calories in 1 cup

Spaghetti with meatballs & tomato sauce	300 calories in 1 cup (some fat)
Oatmeal (cooked)	65 calories in 1/2 cup
Cream of wheat	100 calories 1 cup
Corn flakes	100 calories in 1 cup (some sugar)
Frosted corn flakes	155 calories in 1 cup (sugary)
Shredded Wheat	90 calories in 1 biscuit
Quaker Puffed Rice	120 calories 1 cup (some sugar)
Rice Krispies	110 calories 1 cup (some sugar)
Special K	110 calories 1 cup (some sugar)
Total	110 calories 1 cup (some sugar)
Wheaties	110 calories 1 cup (some sugar)
Cheerios	110 calories 1 cup (some sugar)
Grape Nuts	100 calories 1 cup
Product 19	110 calories 1 cup (some sugar)
Bagel	165 calories in 1 (low fat)
Biscuit	105 calories in 1 (low fat)
Rye bread	60 calories in 1 slice
White bread	70 calories in 1 slice
Whole-wheat bread	65 calories in 1 slice
Hamburger or hot dog bun	120 calories in 1
Cheese pizza	185 calories in 1 medium slice (some fat)
Popcorn	40 calories in 1 cup (low fat)
Pretzel	25 calories in 1
Muffin	120 calories in 1 (low fat, low sugar)
Corn muffin	125 calories in 1 (low fat, low sugar)
Graham crackers	110 calories in 4 (low fat, low sugar)
Saltine crackers	50 calories in 4 (low fat, low sugar)

Cake doughnut (plain)	125 calories in 1 (some fat, some sugar)
Pancake (plain)	60 calories in 1 medium (low fat)
Waffle (plain)	205 calories in 1 (some fat)
Angel food cake	135 calories in 1 medium piece (some sugar)
Cupcake with icing	130 calories in 1 (some fat, sugary)
Chocolate cake	235 calories in 1 piece (some fat, sugary)
Gingerbread	175 calories in 1 piece (low fat, sugary)
Brownie	85 calories in 1 medium (some fat, some sugar)
Chocolate chip cookie	50 calories in 1 cookie (some fat, some sugar)
Apple pie	350 calories in 1 medium piece (fatty, sugary)
Lemon meringue pie	305 calories in 1 medium piece (fatty, sugary)
Pumpkin pie	275 calories in 1 medium piece (fatty, sugary)

Spreads, Sauces & Sweets:

Butter	35 calories in 1 pat (fatty)
Mayonnaise	100 calories in 1 tablespoon (fatty)
French salad dressing	65 calories in 1 tablespoon (fatty)
Syrup	60 calories in 1 tablespoon (sugary)
Honey	80 calories 2 tablespoons (sugary)
Cola	145 calories in 1 can (sugary)
Fudge	115 calories in 1 ounce (some fat, sugary)
Baby Ruth	260 calories 1 bar (fatty, sugary)
Butterfinger	220 calories 1 bar (fatty, sugary)
Hershey's milk chocolate	190 calories 1 bar (fatty, sugary)
Hershey's with almonds	180 calories a bar (fatty, sugary)
Kit Kat	180 calories 1 bar (fatty, sugary)
Kisses	28 calories 1 kiss (fatty, sugary)
Mars	235 calories 1 bar (fatty, sugary)
M & M's Plain	235 calories 1 pkg (fatty, sugary)

M & M's Peanut	240 calories 1 pkg (fatty, sugary)
Snickers	275 calories 1 bar (fatty, sugary)
Three Musketeers	255 calories 1 bar (fatty, sugary)
Tootsie Roll	115 calories 1 bar (fatty, sugary)

FITNESS ON YOUR OWN

If you have the energy and strength to do everyday activities without getting tried or hurt and have energy left for fun and for emergencies, then you are physically fit. The President's Council on Physical Fitness and Sports explains fitness this way: "When you are physically fit, your heart, lungs, and muscles are strong and your body is firm and flexible." A fit person does not have extra fat on the body. The body of a physically fit person is flexible and strong. A fit person's muscles, including the heart, can work for a long time.

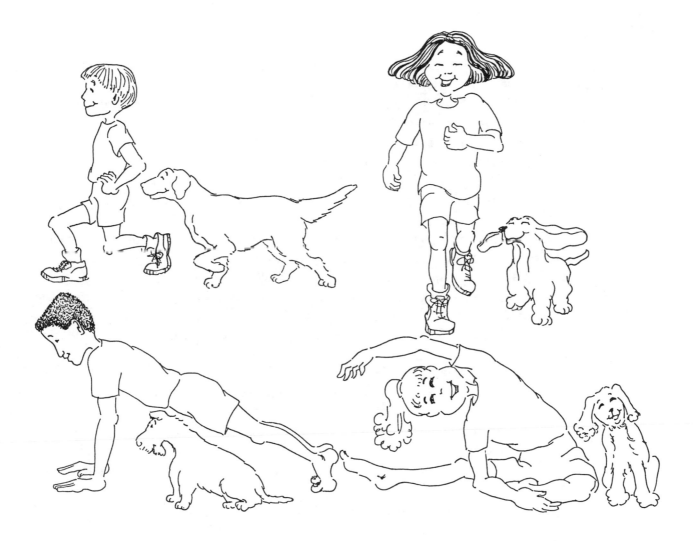

Remember the four types of physical fitness: cardiovascular fitness, muscular strength, muscular endurance, and flexibility? You have been developing all of these parts of fitness during this unit by working out, becoming stronger, and stretching. Now it's time to put all the parts together in your own personal fitness plan.

ACTIVITY: OUTLINING A FITNESS PLAN

With a partner or teammates, you will make a fitness plan during this lesson. In the next two lessons, you will learn how to be active safely and to plan strategies so you will stick with your fitness plan.

Lesson 2 introduced you to the idea of a complete fitness plan. Remember that the order of your exercises and activities makes a difference. A plan should start with exercises that warm up muscles and get joints moving. A plan should include exercises that build muscular strength, muscular endurance, and cardiovascular fitness. The plan should end with cool-down exercises that gradually slow the heart rate and stretch the muscles. You will have a chance to review the information from the previous lessons as you outline your plan.

Procedure

A.   Teammate 1:   Find answers to the following questions about warm-up exercises and about exercises that develop muscular strength.
       This activity will be easier if you work in a team of three. That way you can divide up the questions and finish more quickly. Use all the information in the previous lessons to help you find answers to the questions.
       1.   What is the purpose of warm-up exercises?
       2.   What part or parts of fitness do warm-up exercises improve?
       3.   At what speed do warm-up exercises start? Do they get faster or slower?
       4.   What are two examples of warm-up exercises?
       5.   How would you explain the two principles of specificity and overload to someone who wants to develop muscular strength and endurance?
       6.   What are three major muscle groups you should strengthen?
       7.   What are two examples of exercises that will improve muscular strength and endurance?
B.   Teammate 2: Find answers to the following questions about cardiovascular (aerobic) exercises.
       8.   What is the purpose of cardiovascular (aerobic) exercise?
       9.   What part or parts of fitness do aerobic exercises improve?
       10.   How long should aerobic exercises last?
       11.   Aerobic exercises should raise the pulse rate. Where can you check your pulse rate?
       12.   Give four examples of aerobic activities.
C.   Teammate 3:   Find answers to the following questions about cool-down (flexibility) exercises.
       13.   What is the purpose of cool-down exercises?
       14.   What part or parts of fitness do cool-down exercises improve?
       15.   Should cool-down exercises get faster or slower?
       16.   How should stretching exercises be done (quickly, slowly, smoothly, with bouncing)?
       17.   Give four examples of cool-down exercises.

4. Share your answers with your teammates. Make sure everyone understands and agrees with each answer.

    If you have differences of opinion about an answer, try to find the information in a previous lesson so all teammates can agree.

5. As a team, decide on the order of exercises or activities that go into a fitness plan and write the order on a sheet of paper.

    You answered questions about warm-up exercises, cool-down exercises, exercises that develop muscular strength and endurance, and aerobic exercises. In what order should you put those parts of a fitness plan?

ACTIVITY: MOVE IT!

Procedure

1. Your teacher will assign you and your partner or teammates one component of fitness: warm-up exercises, cardiovascular fitness, muscular strength and endurance, or flexibility.

2. Review your suggestions from questions 2, 7, 12, and 17, depending on the component of fitness your team was assigned.

    For example, if your teacher assigned muscular strength and endurance to your team, you should review your answers to question 7.

3. Prepare to lead the class in the activities or exercises you suggested for your assigned component of fitness.

    Decide who will demonstrate each exercise or activity you chose. Be sure your teacher approves your plan.

4. Participate in a complete workout plan designed by you and your classmates. Be sure you begin with warm-up activities and end with a cool down.

5. Discuss the activities you liked best. Could you do those activities at home?

ACTIVITY: DEVELOPING MY OWN FITNESS PLAN

Now that you and your teammates have researched and practiced what goes into a fitness plan, it's time for you to make one. This needs to be a personal plan, one that you can follow. It should have all the components of fitness, but be organized in a way that is right for you.

Procedure

1. On a sheet of paper, number down the left side from 1 to 10. Leave a couple of lines between each number. After each number, write an activity you like to do that involves movement.

    Your list can include games, sports, individual activities, exercises, walking--anything that gets you moving and using your muscles.

2. Next to each activity, write a "C" if it improves cardiovascular fitness, an "M" if it improves muscular strength or endurance, and an "F" if it improves flexibility.

    You can write more than one letter beside an activity if it improves more than one part of fitness.

3.   Next to each activity, write whether you like to do this activity alone or with someone else. *You can use a code, such as "A" for alone and "WS" for with someone.*

4.   Next, put a * by the three activities you like the best.

5.   Finally, write next to each activity whether you can do this activity from your home or at school or if someone has to take you somewhere special to do this activity.
     Your code could be "No Help" for those activities you can do from home or school. You could use "Help" for those activities that you need some assistance to get to a special location or buy equipment.

6.   Look at your list again. Below your list or on the back of the paper, write what would keep you from doing these activities. Leave a space or two between each reason for not exercising or being active.
     Your reasons could be things like: "My parents won't let me ride my bike very far from home if I am alone. None of my friends like to ride bikes." Or, "It costs money to go skating and I never have enough money." Or, "Sometimes I want to jog around the track at school, but I am too embarrassed to do it by myself."

7.   After each reason for not doing an activity, write something that could motivate you to do the activity.
     Your motivators could be things like: "If I did a couple more chores at home, then my parents might raise my allowance and I would have money to go skating." Or, "If I called my friends ahead of time, one of them would ride bikes with me after school." Try to be realistic about your motivators, but try to get rid of your excuses for not exercising.

8.   Share your lists with a partner or in a team. Compare the things that keep you from exercising and being active. Compare your motivators. Suggest additional motivators that could work for you, your partner, or both of you.

WRAP UP

As a class, make a list of the things you can do to be more active. How can fitness become a regular part of your life? Then, list motivators that might encourage people to be active more often. Get rid of all the excuses and think FITNESS!!

INVOLVING FAMILY MEMBERS

Interview a family member who exercises or works out regularly. (If no one in your family is an active exerciser, then interview a neighbor or relative who is.) Ask about his or her motivators. What keeps that person active? How does he or she find time to exercise on a regular basis? What would he or she advise you to do to become more active?

LESSON 9

SAFETY FIRST

READING: A RIDE TO THE PARK

"What a gorgeous day!" Carol thought as she got up. "How lucky for me that today is Saturday. I can spend the whole day outside."

She called her friend Chet and asked him to go bike riding with her. He agreed, and they decided to ride their bikes to the park.

Carol got ready. First, she checked the tires and brakes on her bike. Then, she told her mother where she was going.

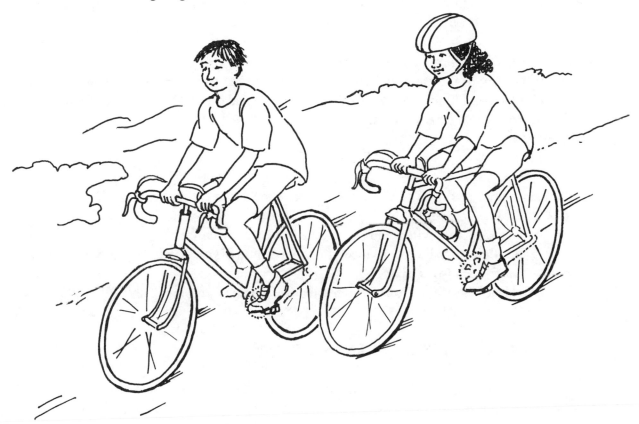

When Chet arrived, Carol put on her helmet and grabbed her water bottle. Chet laughed because he said Carol looked funny wearing the helmet. Carol felt embarrassed. Her mother insisted that she wear it, so she did. She planned to take it off as soon as she got to the park.

As they were cycling, Chet and Carol were caught in a rain shower. It was a light rain, so they continued. When they got to the hill that led to the park, Chet zoomed ahead. He tried to stop for the stop sign at the bottom of the hill, but his wheels skidded on the damp roadway. He fell and hit his head. At first, he just lay there. Then, he sat up in a daze. Blood began to trickle down his face from a cut on his forehead.

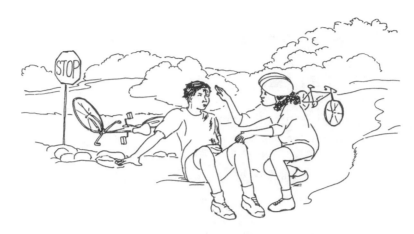

Carol told Chet to stay still. She pressed her hand against his forehead to stop the bleeding. Soon, other people, including Carol's friends Jean and Terry, crowded around to see what happened. Carol asked Jean and Terry to call Chet's parents and ask them to come for him.

As Chet's parents left with Chet and his bike, Carol said, "Hope you feel better soon. Maybe we can get all the way to the park another time." Carol turned to Jean and Terry and said, "Chet thought my helmet looked funny. Now, I'll bet he wishes he had one." Carol and her friends walked to the park and had a great time in the sunshine.

Stop and Discuss

1.   What safety precautions did Carol take before she started riding her bike?
2.   Could Chet have prevented his injury? If so, how?
3.   Do you wear a helmet when you ride a bike? Why or why not?
4.   Did reading this story help convince you to wear one if you don't? What would convince you or your friends to wear one?
5.   Is it difficult to be safe in front of your friends if being safe seems "uncool"? Why or why not?

ACTIVITY: MAKING FITNESS PLANS SAFE

In the previous lesson, you outlined a fitness plan. To carry out your plan and become fit, you need to avoid injuries. In this lesson, you will review your fitness plan and think about ways to do the activities safely.

Procedure

1.   With a partner or in a team, review one another's lists of activities from the previous lesson.
2.   Identify possible hazards in the activities on each list.
        Could you become injured if you didn't wear protective equipment? Could you become injured if you had to ride your bike on a busy street? Could you become injured if you went swimming where there was no lifeguard present? List anything that could result in injuries.

3. Review the reading "Safety Tips for Physical Fitness Activities." Read carefully any section that applies to the activities on any of your team member's lists.

4. Using the information from the reading, write safety tips next to each activity that would make that activity more safe.

    If an activity you have chosen is not part of the reading on safety tips, talk to your teacher or find books in the library that will provide safety tips for that activity.

Stop and Discuss

1. Why should we be concerned about safety in a unit on physical fitness?
2. What would prevent you from taking safety precautions for the activities you like to do?
3. What might encourage you to take safety precautions?

READING: SAFETY TIPS FOR PHYSICAL FITNESS ACTIVITIES

The following readings include safety tips for walking, jogging, bicycling, skateboarding, water sports, rope skipping, and general suggestions about sports safety. Use these tips to help you become fit safely.

A. Safety Tips for Walking

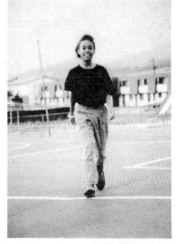

Walking is an excellent aerobic activity. It requires no special equipment, it costs nothing, and most people can walk for 20 or 30 minutes at a time. You can walk almost anywhere, and walking is easier on the joints than jogging. If you decide to walk, you should follow these basic rules for safety and comfort:

1. Let someone know where you are going and when you expect to be back. Choose places without a lot of cars, dogs, or poisonous plants. Also, look for places with flat surfaces without holes.
2. Wear socks and comfortable shoes that have a thick sole.
3. If you walk along roadways, walk facing traffic. Walk as far to the left as possible. Obey traffic rules and signals, and watch for cars.
4. As you walk uphill, lean forward. Going downhill, take shorter steps and straighten up.

5. Before a long walk, drink some water. Carry water with you and drink it often.
6. Walk quickly and try not to stop. Check your pulse. Decide whether you are walking fast enough to reach your target heart rate. Remember to keep moving for at least 20 minutes.
7. Carry some first aid tape with you. If you feel a blister developing, protect the blister with tape.
8. Often, it is not safe to walk at night. If you do, wear light-colored clothing or clothing with reflective strips. Carry a flashlight and never walk alone. Choose familiar, well-lit places.
9. Look around and enjoy the area. Try to find something new every time you walk. Have fun!!

B. Safety Tips for Jogging

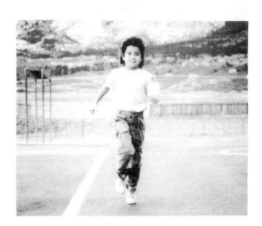

Jogging builds heart and lung endurance better than most exercises. Joggers require no special equipment except proper shoes. Jogging costs nothing once you have the shoes, and you can jog in many places.

Jogging does pound knee, hip, and ankle joints. Sometimes, joggers have soreness in these joints. If you decide to jog, here are some safety tips:

1. Let someone know where you are going and when you expect to be back. Choose places without a lot of cars, dogs, or poisonous plants. Also, look for places with flat surfaces.
2. Wear socks and comfortable shoes that have a thick sole.
3. If you jog along roadways, jog facing traffic. Stay as far to the left as possible. Obey traffic signals and watch for cars.
4. Be sure to warm up before and cool down after jogging.
5. Before jogging, drink some water. If you are going to jog for more than 20 to 30 minutes, plan your course so you can stop to drink water along the way (at a friend's house, a gas station, a park water fountain).
6. Every few minutes, slow down to a walk and check your pulse. Decide whether you are in your target heart-rate zone. If you are breathing so hard you cannot talk, slow down. It is okay to walk for a while.

7.   Carry some first aid tape with you. If you feel a blister developing, protect the blister with tape.

8.   It is not safe to jog at night, especially alone. It is hard to see potholes or other hazards in the roadway. If you do jog at night, wear light-colored clothing or clothing with reflective strips. Always carry a flashlight and never jog alone at night. Jog in familiar, well-lit places.

C. Safety Tips for Bicycling

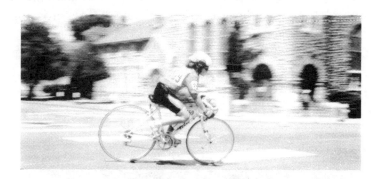

Riding a bike can be fun. You can get places faster on a bike than you can by walking. Riding a bike improves the endurance of your leg muscles. It also exercises your heart and lungs and helps build a lean body.

Follow these tips for safe bicycle riding:

1.   Let someone know where you are going and when you expect to be back.

2.   Be sure your bike is in good working order. Check the following:
     Height of the seat: You should be able to touch the pedals. Your leg should bend only slightly when the pedal is straight down. Your legs cannot work efficiently if the seat is too low. You cannot handle the bike well if the seat is too high. Take your bike to a bicycle store if you are not sure how high the seat should be.
     Brakes: They should stop you. They should not slip or squeal.
     Handlebars, seat, wheels, chain, spokes and reflectors: Tighten any loose parts. Replace any broken or missing parts.
     Tires: They should have good tread. They should have enough air. The amount of air pressure required to inflate the tire properly is stamped on the side of the tire.

3.   Wear a helmet. Most serious injuries from bicycling are head injuries and many of those injuries are very serious. Remember, concrete is much harder than your head.

4.   Obey the same rules of the road that drivers of cars do. Ride on the right side of the road, close to the curb. If you are riding with others, ride single file in a straight line. Use hand signals when you plan to turn or stop. Do not make turns into traffic or ride across crosswalks in front of cars. Remember, a car is much heavier than you and cars cannot always stop quickly. In a collision, you would be the loser.

5.   It is unsafe to ride at night. Drivers cannot see you easily and potholes and other hazards are not easy to see. If you must ride at night, make sure your bicycle has a headlight and a rear reflector. Wear light-colored clothing. Never ride alone at night.

6. Use a horn or bell to warn people and animals that you are approaching. Pedestrians have the right-of-way.

7. Watch for people in parked cars. They may open the door or suddenly pull into traffic.

8. Do not carry riders on your bike. With riders, you cannot see well or handle your bike well. Even an adult should carry a small child only in a special seat behind the rider.

9. Carry packages in a basket, on a rack, or in a backpack, not in your arms.

10. Slow down at intersections. Look both ways before crossing a street. Walk your bike across busy intersections.

Remember, when you ride a bike, you are much less protected than you are in a car. You should be alert at all times. Look, listen, and be smart. If it is raining, be extra careful. Your brakes will not work well on wet roads.

D. Safety Tips for Skateboarding

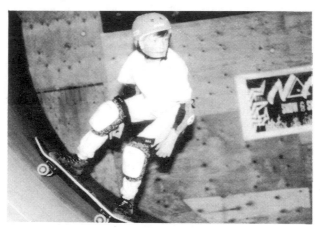

Skateboarding burns calories. It develops muscular endurance in the legs, flexibility, and balance, but it is not a good way to build heart and lung endurance.

Skateboarding can be fun. It can also result in injuries. Here are pointers for safe skateboarding:

1. Let someone know where you will be and when you expect to be back. Skateboard only where it is legal.

2. Do other activities to build fitness before you start skateboarding.

3. Warm up before you start.

4. Wear high-top sneakers that have support and padding. Wear socks and long pants.

5. Wear knee pads and a helmet. Tape your hands or wear gloves.

6. Learn how to fall without injuring yourself.

7. If you skateboard on the street, obey the laws for walkers. Be careful crossing streets. Look for cracks, rocks, and holes.

8. Carry first aid tape with you. If you feel a blister developing, protect the blister with tape.

9.   Be polite to walkers when you are skateboarding. Respect people's property.
10.   Clean and lubricate the bearings of your skateboard regularly--every two weeks if you skateboard often.
11.   Know your limits. Do not try difficult stunts until you can do easier ones.

D. Safety Tips for Water Sports

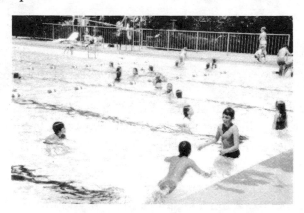

Many people enjoy swimming, boating, and other activities in and around water. Continuous swimming is an excellent aerobic exercise. It can also develop muscular endurance. Because it burns calories, swimming is a good way to develop a lean body. Other activities related to water, such as boating, are not as effective for improving fitness, but they can still be fun.

To stay safe in and around water, follow these tips:

1.   Learn to swim.
2.   Never swim by yourself. Always have a buddy.
3.   Swim only in areas supervised by a lifeguard or another trained person.
4.   Know your limits.
5.   Wear a life preserver in a boat. If you are in a small boat that turns over, stay with the boat if you can.
6.   Use sunscreen to protect yourself from sunburn.
7.   When you start to shiver, get out of the water.
8.   Know the area where you are going to swim. Be sure the water is deep enough before you dive. Be sure there is nothing sticking up from the bottom. Ask a lifeguard if there are any holes or dangerous currents.
9.   Move away from the water when there is lightning in the area.
10.   Do not run on pool decks. Do not use glass containers around pools or on beaches. Do not push people into the water or hold them under.
11.   Do not go anywhere on a raft where it would be unsafe to swim.
12.   Be sure ice is at least four inches thick before skating on a pond or lake.

There are many sports you can play with others. Basketball, soccer, softball, hockey, and flag football are some favorites. Each has its own fitness benefits. Many people like the chance to be with other people.

Each sport has its own rules, but there are some general safety tips for all sports:

1. Learn the rules of the game.
2. Practice the skills you need.
3. Wear the suggested protective equipment and proper shoes.
4. Get in shape before you play.
5. Warm up before playing. Cool down afterward.
6. While playing, drink a lot of water, especially if it is hot and humid.
7. Don't overdo. Injuries happen when you are tired and your muscles are fatigued.
8. Do not play if you have an injury. Let an injury heal completely before you participate again.
9. Learn to play as a team rather than as a group of individuals.
10. Enjoy the sport, whether you win or lose.

WRAP UP

Debate whether your state should have safety laws requiring

- bicycle helmets;
- motorcycle helmets;
- mouth guards for sports such as football, hockey, and soccer;
- knee pads for skateboarding;
- lifeguards for all swimming areas (including apartment and hotel pools) that are open to the public; and
- life preservers on all boats.

INVOLVING FAMILY MEMBERS

Share the safety tips with family members and encourage them to wear helmets when they bicycle, wear proper shoes when they walk or jog, and wear protective equipment and mouth guards when they play sports. Make a contract with your family to play it safe at all times.

LESSON 10

BECOMING FIT

ACTIVITY: MAKING A FITNESS PLAN

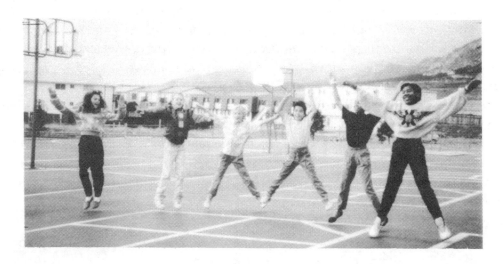

Your fitness plan is meant to be a personal plan for you. Plan to make a commitment for at least one week. When you fill in your chart, choose activities you know you could be excited about making a part of your life. Be realistic. Think about the weather, the cost, and the positive health benefits. This could be one of the best things you have ever done for yourself. Good luck and have fun becoming fit.

Procedure

1.   Review your list from Lesson 8 of the 10 activities you like to do. As you look over your activities, ask yourself these questions:
    a.   Have I included activities that will improve all four parts of fitness?
    b.   Have I included activities that will make my heart beat faster for at least 15 minutes?
    c.   Have I chosen activities I really like to do?
    d.   Have I involved my friends or my family in my activities?
2.   Make a blank fitness plan chart like the one shown below.

MY FITNESS PLAN

Day	Warm-up Activities	Aerobic Activities	Strength Activities	Cool-down Activities	When?	Where?	With Whom?

3.   Look at your list from Lesson 8. Which activities would work for warm-up, muscular strength, aerobic (cardiovascular) fitness, and cool-down (flexibility)? Write the activities in the first four columns.

Write the activities in pencil because you might change your mind about which activities you want to do on different days of the week once you look at your whole plan. You can also write one activity in more than one box if it is something you like to do often.

4.   Fill in the boxes in your chart that are blank. What other activities might you include? Write **when** you will exercise, **where** you will exercise, and **with whom**.

You may work with a partner to complete your fitness chart. You can suggest activities or exercises to one another. You can help one another decide when you would be likely to exercise, where, and with whom. Remember, you do not have to work on all components of fitness every day.

5.   Once you have filled in all the boxes, look over each person's fitness plan and identify ways to help one another succeed.

If you want to do some activities that you are unable to do, ask your partner for help. Maybe together you can figure out ways to help you overcome the problems. Sometimes, people get discouraged after a short time because they do not see any changes. Think of ways you and your partner can encourage each other if one of you gets discouraged.

6.   Show your chart to your teacher for approval.

7.   As a class, decide how you could reward one another for following your plans.

WRAP UP

Check in with your classmates every day during the week. Find out which of you followed your fitness plans the previous day. Congratulate those who did. Encourage those who had problems or are giving up, and help one another find ways to overcome these problems. Try to get everyone to continue with their plans.

Talk about any changes you decided to make. Did you find activities that you like better? Did a friend invite you to do something that was more fun than what you had in your plan?

Discuss the results of your fitness activities. Do you feel better after exercising? Do you think you will become more active on a regular basis? Why or why not?

Your fitness level probably will not change in just one week, but trying to set aside time for fitness will help you change your life for lifelong fitness. If you keep with it, you will notice changes in how you feel and how you look. Keep up the good work that you have started!

INVOLVING FAMILY MEMBERS

Make a fitness plan as a family. What activities could you do together? You might make plans to do something simple like walking together or you could plan more elaborate activities like going on hikes or participating on community teams through the parks and recreation department. The important goal is to get up off the couch, turn off the television, and get moving! Even if you are active for only 20 to 30 minutes each day, you will be on your way to feeling good and looking good.